Contents

Crepes 11
Sausage Gravy and Biscuits 11
Western Frittata 12
Pumpkin Crumb Muffins 12
Breakfast Burritos 13
Easy Apple Cinnamon Crumb Muffins 14
Bacon and Egg Muffins 15
Cinnamon Roll French Toast Casserole 16
Cinnamon Roll Muffins 17
Baked Pumpkin Donuts 18
Shakshuka 19
Apple Cinnamon Baked Oatmeal Cups 19
Sausage Balls 20
Sausage Hash Brown Egg Cups 20
Banana Nut Muffins 21
Breakfast Cookies 21
Country Breakfast Skillet 22
Baked Apple Cinnamon Donuts 23
Turkey Sausage Patties 23
Classic French Toast 24
Grilled Chicken Chimichurri Salad 24
Smoked Salmon Sushi Bowls 25
Asian Chicken Lettuce Wraps 26
Creamy Italian Pasta Salad 27
Tuna Salad Avocado Bowls 28
Southern Chicken Salad 28
Taco Salad 29
Soy Ginger Vegetable Stir-Fry 29
Southwest Tricolored Quinoa Salad 30
Avocado Bacon Chicken Salad 31

Southwestern Chicken Salad	31
Chopped Asian Salad with Peanut Dressing	32
Egg Roll Bowl	33
Homestyle Egg Salad	33
Greek Chicken Wraps	34
Mediterranean Tuna Salad	34
Mini Corn Dog Bites	35
Spinach Salad with Warm Bacon Dressing	35
Crispy Southwest Wraps	36
Loaded Burger Bowls	37
Grilled Chicken Caesar Salad	38
Grilled Chicken Cobb Salad	39
Broiled Romaine Salad with Balsamic Glaze	40
Sloppy Joe Baked Potatoes	40
Traditional Greek Salad	41
Spinach and Artichoke Chicken	41
Crispy Baked Barbecue Chicken Thighs	42
Paleo Pesto Turkey Meatballs	43
Crunchy Coconut Chicken Bites	43
Turmeric Coconut Chicken Curry	44
Asian Apricot Chicken	44
Oven-Fried Chicken	45
Chicken and Dumplings Casserole	46
Moroccan Chicken	47
Chicken Alfredo	47
Chicken Piccata	48
Tuscan Chicken	49
Crispy Baked Chicken Thighs	50
Rosemary Roasted Chicken	50
Honey Garlic Chicken	50
Chicken Scaloppine	51
Baked Balsamic Chicken	52

Sesame Chicken 52
Savory Roasted Milk Chicken Thighs 53
Hawaiian Chicken Kebabs 54
Teriyaki Chicken 55
Baked Honey Mustard Chicken 55
Pasta Primavera with Chicken 56
Chicken and Dumplings 57
Buffalo Turkey Burgers 57
Easy Chicken Fried Rice 58
Chicken Marsala 58
Melt-in-Your-Mouth Chicken Breasts 59
Easy Homemade Chicken Nuggets 59
Baked Bacon Ranch Chicken Breasts 60
Chicken Fajitas 61
Bruschetta Chicken Bake 61
Homestyle Chicken and Rice Casserole 62
Honey Lemon Ginger Chicken 63
Easy Baked Lemon Pepper Chicken 63
Southern Chicken-Fried Steak 64
Mongolian Beef 65
Brown Butter Filet Mignon 65
Cottage Pie 66
Mini Meatloaves 66
Sautéed Beef with Broccoli 67
Swedish Meatballs 68
Easy Homemade Beef Stroganoff 68
Stuffed Peppers 69
Salisbury Steak 70
Oven-Baked St. Louis–Style Ribs 71
Beef Tenderloin 71
Prime Rib 72
Easy Bacon Burger Pie 73

Taco Beef	73
Korean Beef	74
Pork Chop Suey	74
Italian Meatballs	75
Southwestern Tamale Pie	75
Baked Ham with Brown Sugar Glaze	76
Pork Tenderloin	77
Smothered Pork Chops	77
German Pork Chops	78
Honey Garlic Pork Chops	79
Sweet and Sour Pork	79
Crispy Salmon Cakes	80
Cajun Catfish	81
Fish Tacos	82
Classic Shrimp Scampi	82
Maryland-Style Crab Cakes	83
Country Shrimp and Grits	84
Honey Soy–Glazed Salmon	84
Steamed Mussels with Marsala Wine and Garlic	85
Cajun Jambalaya	85
Stuffed Jumbo Shrimp	86
Lemon Garlic Sautéed Scallops	87
Baked Salmon with Lemon	88
Cilantro Lime Shrimp Bake	88
Clams Casino	89
New England Clam Bake	89
Oven-Fried Orange Roughy	90
Grilled Grouper with Lemon Butter Sauce	90
Pecan-Crusted Honey Mustard Salmon	91
Chili Lime Tilapia with Fresh Mango Salsa	91
Marinated Grilled Tuna Steaks	92
Greek-Style Snapper	93

New Orleans–Style Barbecue Shrimp	93
Spaghetti with White Clam Sauce	94
Curried Shrimp	94
Crispy Baked Fish Sticks	95
Roasted Garlic Potatoes	96
Easy Rice Pilaf	96
Baked Sweet Potato Fries	96
Balsamic-Roasted Brussels Sprouts	97
Ratatouille	98
Creamy Scalloped Potatoes	98
Potato Pancakes	99
Honey-Glazed Carrots	99
Southwestern Black Bean and Corn Salad	100
Cheesy Green Bean Casserole	100
Italian Roasted Vegetables	101
Roasted Butternut Squash	101
Sautéed Garlic Green Beans	102
Zucchini Noodles	102
Easy Oven-Roasted Corn on the Cob	102
Southern-Style Sweet Potato Casserole	103
Bacon and Tomato Macaroni Salad	103
Loaded Bacon Ranch Potato Salad	104
Savory Stuffing	104
Easy Homemade Gravy	105
Creamy Dill Sauce	105
Homemade Buttermilk Ranch Dressing	106
Homemade Honey Mustard Dressing	106
Balsamic Vinaigrette Salad Dressing	106
Homemade Tartar Sauce	107
Bread Machine Bread	107
Easy One-Bowl Banana Bread	108
Double Chocolate Banana Bread	108

Soft Homemade Dinner Rolls	109
Easy Thick-Crust Pizza Dough	110
Chocolate Chip Quick Bread	111
Southern Sweet Corn Bread	111
Apple Cinnamon Quick Bread	112
Southern Buttermilk Biscuits	112
Lemon Blueberry Scones	113
Jam-Filled Danish	114
Cinnamon Biscuits	115
Homemade Bagels	116
Rosemary Focaccia Bread	117
Soft Pretzels	118
Flatbread	119
Homemade Popovers	120
Herbed Crusty Bread	120
Lemon Blueberry Quick Bread	121
Garlic Breadsticks	122
Marbled Quick Bread	122
Potato Rolls	123
Cranberry Orange Quick Bread	124
Cream of Mushroom Soup	124
Savory Chicken and Rice Soup	125
Loaded Baked Potato Soup	126
Creamy Chicken Corn Chowder	126
Zuppa Toscana	127
Cream of Chicken Soup	128
Hearty Hamburger Soup	128
Italian Vegetable Soup	129
Southern Ham and Bean Soup	129
Chicken Fajita Soup	130
French Onion Soup	131
Classic Tomato Soup	131

Butternut Squash Soup	131
Ramen Soup with Eggs	132
Taco Soup	132
Maryland-Style Cream of Crab Soup	133
White Chicken Chili	134
New England Clam Chowder	134
Mexican Pork Posole	135
Stuffed Pepper Soup	135
Maple Bacon Sweet Potato Soup	136
Black Bean Soup	137
Chicken Pot Pie Soup	137
Egg Drop Soup	138
Tex-Mex Chicken Noodle Soup	138
Crispy Baked Buffalo Wings	139
Fried Green Tomatoes	140
Avocado Spring Rolls with Cashew and Cilantro Dipping Sauce	141
Smoked Salmon Dip	142
Easy Guacamole	142
Deep-Dish Pizza Bites	143
Spinach, Sundried Tomatoes, and Artichoke Dip	143
Sticky Asian Wings	144
Loaded Mashed Potato Bites	145
Party Meatballs	145
Buffalo Chicken Dip	146
Southwestern Queso Dip	146
Buffalo Chicken Bites	147
Chili Lime Bacon-Wrapped Shrimp	147
Fried Pickles	148
Mexican Street Corn Dip	148
Easy Homemade Hummus	149
Seven-Layer Dip	149
Southwestern Spring Rolls	150

Thai Chicken Skewers with Peanut Sauce	151
Italian Bruschetta	151
Smoked Salmon with Cucumber and Dill	152
Classic Deviled Eggs	152
Pico de Gallo	153
Stuffed Mushrooms	153
Pressure Cooker Mexican Rice	154
Pressure Cooker Collard Greens	154
Slow Cooker Black Beans	155
Slow Cooker Apples and Cinnamon	155
Slow Cooker Pork Roast with Savory Gravy	156
Pressure Cooker Baked Potatoes	156
Pressure Cooker Mashed Potatoes	157
Pressure Cooker New Orleans–Style Red Beans and Rice	157
Pressure Cooker Whole Roasted Chicken	158
Pressure Cooker Hard-Boiled Eggs	159
Pressure Cooker Cashew Chicken	159
Pressure Cooker Steak Sandwich	160
Slow Cooker Southern-Style Pinto Beans	161
Pressure Cooker Sweet Potatoes	161
Texas-Style Slow Cooker Beef Chili	162
Rotisserie-Style Shredded Chicken	162
Pressure Cooker Barbecue Pulled Pork	163
Pressure Cooker Chicken Cacciatore	164
Pressure Cooker Corned Beef and Cabbage	165
Slow Cooker Beef Tips and Gravy	166
Pressure Cooker Indian Butter Chicken	166
Slow Cooker Pot Roast with Savory Gravy	167
Pressure Cooker Chicken, Broccoli, and Rice	168
Slow Cooker Lemon Garlic Chicken	169
Slow Cooker Orange Chicken	169
Chocolate Chip Cookies	170

Fluffy Sugar Cookies	171
The Perfect Pie Crust	171
Butter Pound Cake	172
Fudgy Brownies	173
Classic Vanilla Cake with Chocolate Buttercream	173
Cinnamon Roll Cake	174
Pumpkin Bread Cookies	175
Apple Bundt Cake	176
Peanut Butter Cookies	177
Pineapple Upside Down Cake	178
Carrot Cake with Cream Cheese Frosting	179
Better Than Banana Bread Cookies	180
Dutch Apple Pie	181
Cowboy Cookies	182
Cinnamon Apple Fries	182
White Cake with Almond Vanilla Buttercream	183
Strawberry Cupcakes with Strawberry Buttercream Frosting	184
Lemon Crinkle Cookies	185
Double Chocolate Chip Cookies	186
Mini "Cheesecakes"	186
Old-Fashioned Oatmeal Raisin Cookies	187
Apple Crisp	188
Pistachio Cookies	189
Coconut Cream Pie	190
Hummingbird Cake with Cream Cheese Frosting	190
Red Velvet Cookies	192
Chocolate-Covered Coconut Macaroons	192
Easy Gluten-Free Chocolate Cake with Chocolate Buttercream Frosting	193
Chocolate Peanut Butter Brownies	195
Frosted Coconut Cake	195
Cinnamon Roll Cookies	196
Apple Pie Blondies	198

Peanut Butter Blossoms..199

Crepes

- **Ingredients :**
- 2 large eggs
- ¾ cup unsweetened almond milk
- ½ cup water
- 1 cup gluten-free all-purpose flour without xanthan gum
- ¼ teaspoon xanthan gum
- 2 tablespoons granulated sugar
- 1 teaspoon pure vanilla extract
- 3 tablespoons dairy-free buttery spread, melted

Directions :

1. In a large bowl, whisk eggs with a mixer. Add remaining ingredients and mix on medium for 1 minute until combined and batter is smooth.

2. Spray a crepe pan with gluten-free nonstick cooking spray. Pour ¼ cup batter into the center of the pan. Pick up the pan and swirl it to spread batter evenly. Cook over medium heat for 30–45 seconds or until browned on the bottom. Flip the crepe over and cook for about 30 more seconds until brown on the other side. Repeat with remaining batter.

3. Slide the crepe onto a plate, laying it flat. Serve crepes rolled or folded into triangles.

Sausage Gravy and Biscuits

- **Ingredients :**
- 1 pound gluten-free ground sausage
- 1 tablespoon garlic powder
- 1 tablespoon onion powder
- 2 cups unsweetened almond milk
- 4 tablespoons gluten-free all-purpose flour with xanthan gum
- 1 teaspoon salt
- 1 teaspoon ground black pepper
- 2 tablespoons dairy-free buttery spread

Directions :

1. In a large skillet, combine sausage, garlic powder, and onion powder. Cook over medium heat for 3–5 minutes, stirring often, until sausage is browned and crumbled.

2. In a small bowl, whisk milk, flour, salt, and pepper for 1 minute until the flour dissolves. Pour the milk mixture into the skillet and cook for 10 minutes, stirring as it thickens. Stir in buttery spread.

3. Serve over biscuits.

Western Frittata

- **Ingredients :**
- 2 tablespoons olive oil
- ½ cup seeded and diced green bell pepper
- ½ cup seeded and diced red bell pepper
- ½ cup peeled and diced sweet onion
- 1½ cups diced cooked gluten-free, dairy-free ham
- 12 large eggs
- ¼ cup unsweetened almond milk
- ½ teaspoon salt

Directions :

1. Preheat oven to 425°F.

2. Add olive oil, bell peppers, onions, and ham to a 12" oven-safe skillet. Cook over medium-high heat for 2–3 minutes until vegetables are tender.

3. Add eggs in a medium bowl and whisk until the whites and yolks are combined. (Do not overmix; whisk only enough to blend the whites and yolks.) Add milk and salt and mix until combined.

4. Pour egg mixture over vegetables. Stir with a spatula to combine and distribute the mixture evenly in the pan.

5. Cook for 1 minute on the stovetop until the edges of the frittata turn lighter in color. Place frittata in the oven and bake for 7–14 minutes until eggs puff up. Remove frittata from the oven and allow to cool for 5–10 minutes before cutting and serving.

Pumpkin Crumb Muffins

Ingredients :

MUFFINS
- 1½ cups canned pumpkin
- 1 teaspoon baking soda
- ¼ cup light brown sugar, packed
- ¼ cup granulated sugar
- 1 tablespoon pumpkin pie spice
- 1 teaspoon ground cinnamon
- ¼ teaspoon salt
- 2 large eggs, room temperature
- 1 teaspoon pure vanilla extract
- 1½ cups gluten-free all-purpose flour with xanthan gum
- ½ teaspoon gluten-free baking powder

- ⅓ cup dairy-free buttery spread, melted

CRUMB TOPPING
- ¼ cup light brown sugar, packed
- 2 tablespoons granulated sugar
- ½ teaspoon pumpkin pie spice
- ⅓ cup gluten-free all-purpose flour with xanthan gum
- 2 tablespoons dairy-free buttery spread, melted

VANILLA MAPLE GLAZE
- 1 cup confectioners' sugar
- 1 teaspoon pure vanilla extract
- 2 tablespoons pure maple syrup
- 1½ teaspoons unsweetened almond milk

Directions :

1. Preheat oven to 350°F. Prepare one twelve-cup muffin tin and two wells of a 6-cup muffin tin with baking cup liners or gluten-free nonstick cooking spray.

2. In a large bowl, add pumpkin, baking soda, brown sugar, granulated sugar, pumpkin pie spice, cinnamon, and salt and mix until ingredients are fully combined. Add eggs and vanilla extract and mix until fully combined.

3. Add flour and baking powder to a small bowl, give it a quick stir, and then pour into the pumpkin mixture. Pour buttery spread into muffin batter and mix until fully combined. The muffin batter will be thick. Scoop batter into prepared muffin tins.

4. To make the crumb topping, add brown sugar, granulated sugar, pumpkin pie spice, and flour to a small bowl and stir until fully combined. Pour in buttery spread and stir until topping looks thick and crumbly. Sprinkle 1 tablespoon of crumb topping on top of each muffin.

5. Bake for 20–25 minutes or until a toothpick inserted in the center of a muffin comes out clean. Place muffin tin on a cooling rack and cool for 2 minutes. Remove muffins from tin and place on rack to continue cooling.

6. In a small bowl, add the glaze ingredients and stir until smooth. Drizzle glaze over tops of muffins. Store in an airtight container for up to 3 days.

Breakfast Burritos

- **Ingredients :**
- 2 tablespoons olive oil
- ½ pound gluten-free ground sausage
- ¼ teaspoon ground cumin
- 4 large eggs

- ¼ teaspoon salt
- 4 gluten-free and dairy-free flour tortillas
- ¼ cup gluten-free salsa
- 1 cup frozen Tater Tots, cooked
- 1 large avocado, peeled, pitted, and diced
- ¼ cup chopped fresh cilantro

Directions :

1. Heat olive oil in a large skillet over medium-high heat. Add sausage and cumin and cook for 5–8 minutes until it is browned and in crumbles. Drain excess oil, reserving 1 tablespoon in the skillet.

2. Whisk eggs and salt in a small bowl and add to the sausage in the skillet. Reduce heat to low and scramble for 2–3 minutes until just cooked through.

3. Heat each tortilla in a medium pan over medium heat for 1–2 minutes or in the microwave for 10–15 seconds.

4. Spread salsa down the center of each tortilla. Top with Tater Tots, sausage, eggs, avocado, and cilantro, then roll the burrito.

Easy Apple Cinnamon Crumb Muffins

Ingredients :

MUFFINS
- 1½ cups unsweetened applesauce
- ⅓ cup dairy-free buttery spread, melted
- 2 large eggs, room temperature
- ½ cup granulated sugar
- ⅛ teaspoon salt
- 1 teaspoon pure vanilla extract
- 1½ cups gluten-free all-purpose flour with xanthan gum
- 1 teaspoon baking soda
- ½ teaspoon gluten-free baking powder
- 1 tablespoon ground cinnamon

CRUMB TOPPING
- ¼ cup light brown sugar, packed
- 2 tablespoons granulated sugar
- ½ teaspoon ground cinnamon
- ⅓ cup gluten-free all-purpose flour with xanthan gum
- 2 tablespoons dairy-free buttery spread, melted

Directions :

1. Preheat oven to 350°F. Prepare a twelve-cup muffin tin with baking cup liners or gluten-free nonstick cooking spray.

2. In a large bowl, add applesauce, buttery spread, and eggs and mix together until combined. Stir in granulated sugar, salt, and vanilla extract. Stir in flour, baking soda, baking powder, and cinnamon, and mix until all ingredients are smooth and fully combined.

3. Scoop batter into prepared muffin tin.

4. To make the crumb topping, add brown sugar, granulated sugar, cinnamon, and flour to a small bowl and stir until fully combined. Pour in buttery spread and stir until the topping looks thick and crumbly. Sprinkle 1 tablespoon of crumb topping on top of each muffin.

5. Bake for 20 minutes or until a toothpick inserted in the center comes out clean. Place muffin tin on a cooling rack and cool for 2 minutes. Remove muffins from tin and place on rack to finish cooling. Store in an airtight container at room temperature for up to 3 days.

Bacon and Egg Muffins

- **Ingredients :**
- 2 cups gluten-free all-purpose flour with xanthan gum
- ¼ cup sugar
- 1 tablespoon gluten-free baking powder
- ½ teaspoon baking soda
- ½ teaspoon salt
- 2 large eggs
- 1 tablespoon white vinegar
- 1 cup unsweetened almond milk
- 1 cup dairy-free buttery spread, melted
- 1 cup chopped cooked gluten-free bacon, divided
- 1 green onion, diced
- 2 large hard-boiled eggs, chopped

Directions :

1. Preheat oven to 375°F. Prepare a twelve-cup muffin tin with baking cup liners or gluten-free nonstick cooking spray.

2. In a large bowl, add flour, sugar, baking powder, baking soda, and salt. Stir to combine. Add uncooked eggs to the flour mixture and mix until fully combined.

3. In a small bowl, add vinegar and milk and let sit for 1–2 minutes.

4. Add buttery spread and the vinegar mixture to batter and mix until fully combined.

5. Reserve 2 tablespoons bacon Add the rest of the bacon, green onions, and hard-boiled eggs to batter. Stir to fully mix everything.

6. Scoop batter into prepared muffin tin. Sprinkle the reserved bacon on top of each muffin.

7. Bake for 30 minutes or until a toothpick inserted in the center of a muffin comes out clean. Place muffin tin on a cooling rack and cool for 2 minutes. Remove muffins from tin and place on rack to finish cooling.

Cinnamon Roll French Toast Casserole

Ingredients :

CASSEROLE
- 1 (14-ounce) loaf gluten-free and dairy-free bread, cut into 1" pieces
- ½ cup light brown sugar
- 1 tablespoon plus 1 teaspoon ground cinnamon, divided
- 6 large eggs, beaten
- 2 cups unsweetened almond milk
- ½ cup granulated sugar
- 1 tablespoon pure vanilla extract

CRUMB TOPPING
- 1 cup gluten-free all-purpose flour with xanthan gum
- ½ cup light brown sugar, packed
- ¼ teaspoon salt
- 1 teaspoon ground cinnamon
- ½ cup dairy-free buttery spread, melted

GLAZE
- 2 cups confectioners' sugar
- 1 teaspoon pure vanilla extract
- 2 tablespoons unsweetened almond milk

Directions :

1. Preheat oven to 350°F. Spray a 9" × 13" baking dish with gluten-free nonstick cooking spray.

2. Spread bread pieces evenly on an ungreased baking sheet and bake for 5–10 minutes until nicely toasted. Remove from the oven when toasted and set aside.

3. In a small bowl, mix together brown sugar and 1 tablespoon cinnamon. Sprinkle the brown sugar mixture on the bottom of the prepared pan. Add the toasted bread pieces over the top of the brown sugar mixture.

4. In a medium bowl, whisk together eggs, milk, granulated sugar, vanilla extract, and remaining 1 teaspoon cinnamon until well blended. Pour the egg mixture evenly over the bread pieces.

5. To make the topping: In a small bowl, add flour, brown sugar, salt, cinnamon, and buttery spread and mix until crumbly. Sprinkle the crumb mixture evenly over the top of the casserole.

6. Bake on the middle rack for 1 hour or until a toothpick inserted in the center comes out clean.

7. Mix the glaze ingredients together in a small bowl until smooth. Allow casserole to cool a few minutes before drizzling glaze on it and serving.

Cinnamon Roll Muffins

Ingredients :

MUFFINS
- 1½ cups gluten-free all-purpose flour with xanthan gum
- ⅛ teaspoon salt
- ½ cup granulated sugar
- 2 teaspoons gluten-free baking powder
- ¾ cup unsweetened almond milk
- 1 large egg
- 1 teaspoon pure vanilla extract
- ¼ cup dairy-free buttery spread, melted

TOPPING
- ¼ cup dairy-free buttery spread, softened
- ¼ cup light brown sugar, packed
- ½ tablespoon gluten-free all-purpose flour with xanthan gum
- ¾ teaspoon ground cinnamon

GLAZE
- 1 cup confectioners' sugar
- 2½ tablespoons unsweetened almond milk
- ½ teaspoon pure vanilla extract

Directions :

1. Preheat oven to 350°F. Prepare a twelve-cup muffin tin with baking cup liners or gluten-free nonstick cooking spray.

2. In a large bowl, add flour, salt, granulated sugar, baking powder, milk, egg, and vanilla and mix until fully combined. Stir in melted buttery spread. Scoop batter into prepared muffin tin.

3. In a separate large bowl, cream the topping ingredients together to make the topping.

4. Drop a teaspoonful of topping on each muffin. Use a knife to swirl the mixture through each muffin.

5. Bake for 20–25 minutes or until a toothpick inserted in the center of a muffin comes out clean. Place muffin tin on a cooling rack and cool for 2 minutes. Remove muffins from tin and place on rack to

continue cooling.

6. In a medium bowl, whisk the glaze ingredients together. Drizzle over warm muffins. Store in an airtight container for up to 3 days.

Baked Pumpkin Donuts

Ingredients :

DONUTS
- ¾ cup sugar
- 2 large eggs, room temperature
- 4 tablespoons vegetable oil
- 1 cup canned pumpkin purée
- 1 teaspoon pure vanilla extract
- 1½ cups gluten-free all-purpose flour with xanthan gum
- ½ teaspoon salt
- 1 teaspoon pumpkin pie spice
- ½ teaspoon ground cinnamon
- 1 teaspoon gluten-free baking powder

GLAZE
- 1 cup confectioners' sugar
- ¼ teaspoon ground cinnamon
- 1 teaspoon pure vanilla extract
- 4 tablespoons pure maple syrup

Directions :

1. Preheat oven to 350°F. Spray a full-sized twelve-cup donut pan with gluten-free nonstick cooking spray.

2. In a large bowl, combine sugar, eggs, vegetable oil, pumpkin purée, and vanilla extract. Mix until fully combined.

3. Add flour, salt, pumpkin pie spice, cinnamon, and baking powder and mix until fully combined. The batter will be thick and sticky.

4. Add batter to a large plastic storage bag or piping bag. Seal the bag and cut a corner (or tip if using a piping bag) off. Carefully squeeze batter into donut pan. Bake for 14–16 minutes until golden brown and set. Place pan on a cooling rack and cool for 1 minute. Remove donuts from the pan and place on rack to continue cooling.

5. In a small bowl, whisk together the glaze ingredients. Dip each warm donut into the glaze and place on a plate or wire rack. Store in an airtight container for up to 3 days.

Shakshuka

- **Ingredients :**
- 3 tablespoons olive oil
- 1 large yellow onion, peeled and chopped
- 2 large green bell peppers, seeded and chopped
- 1 tablespoon jarred minced garlic
- 1 teaspoon ground coriander
- 1 teaspoon paprika
- ½ teaspoon ground cumin
- 1 (28-ounce) can whole peeled tomatoes, including liquid
- ½ teaspoon salt
- ¼ teaspoon ground black pepper
- 1 teaspoon granulated sugar
- 6 large eggs
- ¼ cup chopped fresh cilantro

Directions :

1. In a large skillet, heat olive oil over medium heat. Add onions and bell peppers and sauté for 5 minutes until onions become translucent. Stir in garlic and spices and cook for an additional minute until fragrant.

2. Pour in tomatoes and their juice and break down tomatoes using a spoon. Add salt, black pepper, and sugar and bring the sauce to a simmer.

3. Use a large spoon to make six small wells in the sauce and crack an egg into each well. Cover the skillet and cook for 5–8 minutes or until the eggs are poached to your liking. Spoon an egg and sauce on each plate and serve warm. Garnish with chopped cilantro.

Apple Cinnamon Baked Oatmeal Cups

- **Ingredients :**
- 2 large bananas, peeled and mashed
- 2 large eggs, whisked
- 1 tablespoon pure vanilla extract
- ¼ cup honey
- 2 cups gluten-free oatmeal
- ¼ teaspoon salt
- 1 tablespoon plus ½ teaspoon ground cinnamon, divided
- ⅔ cup unsweetened almond milk
- 1 cup diced Gala apple, divided
- ½ teaspoon lemon juice

Directions :

1. Preheat oven to 400°. Prepare a twelve-cup muffin tin with baking cup liners or gluten-free nonstick cooking spray.
2. In a large bowl, combine bananas, eggs, vanilla, and honey. Stir in gluten-free oatmeal, salt, and 1 tablespoon cinnamon. Add milk and stir.
3. Add chopped apples to a small bowl and toss with ½ teaspoon cinnamon and lemon juice. Add half of apple mixture to batter and stir to combine.
4. Scoop batter into muffin tin and top with remaining apple mixture. Bake for 20 minutes. Allow to cool for 1–2 minutes before serving.

Sausage Balls

Ingredients :
- 3 cups Bisquick Gluten Free Pancake & Baking Mix
- 2 tablespoons dried sage
- 1 tablespoon paprika
- 4 cups shredded dairy-free Cheddar cheese
- 1 cup dairy-free Parmesan cheese
- ½ cup light brown sugar, packed
- 1½ cups unsweetened almond milk
- 2 (16-ounce) packages gluten-free sausage rolls

Directions :
1. Heat oven to 350°F. Line a baking sheet with parchment paper.
2. In a large bowl, mix Bisquick, sage, paprika, cheeses, and brown sugar together. Add milk and stir until fully combined. Add sausage and stir to combine.
3. Using a teaspoon or cookie scoop, make nine dozen 1" balls. Place on prepared baking sheet.
4. Bake for 20–25 minutes until golden brown. Allow to cool for 2–3 minutes before serving.

Sausage Hash Brown Egg Cups

Ingredients :
- 1 teaspoon olive oil
- ½ pound gluten-free ground sausage
- 36 frozen Tater Tots
- 1 teaspoon salt, divided
- 8 large eggs
- 2 tablespoons unsweetened almond milk

Directions :
1. Preheat oven to 400°F and spray a twelve-cup muffin tin with gluten-free nonstick cooking spray.

2. Heat olive oil in a large skillet over medium-high heat. Add sausage and cook for 10 minutes until sausage is crumbly, evenly browned, and no longer pink; drain.

3. Microwave Tater Tots for 1–2 minutes to defrost and soften. Place three Tater Tots in each well of prepared muffin tin. Press down to make a crust and sprinkle a little salt in each well, making sure a pinch of salt is left over.

4. Bake for 10 minutes, then remove from the oven and lower the oven temperature to 350°F.

5. In a medium bowl, whisk eggs and remaining salt. Add milk and combine.

6. Sprinkle sausage on top of Tater Tots. Pour the egg mixture on top of sausage. Bake for 20 minutes. Allow to cool for 2 minutes before removing cups from muffin tin. Serve warm.

Banana Nut Muffins

Ingredients :
- 2 large ripe bananas, peeled and mashed
- 1 teaspoon baking soda
- ⅓ cup dairy-free buttery spread, melted
- ½ cup sugar
- ⅛ teaspoon salt
- 2 large eggs, whisked
- 1 teaspoon pure vanilla extract
- 1½ cups gluten-free all-purpose flour with xanthan gum
- ½ teaspoon ground cinnamon
- ½ cup chopped walnuts

Directions :

1. Preheat oven to 350°F. Prepare a twelve-cup muffin tin with baking cup liners or gluten-free nonstick cooking spray.

2. In a large bowl, combine bananas and baking soda. Allow the mixture to sit for at least 2 minutes. (Allowing the mashed bananas and baking soda to sit for at least 2 minutes before adding the rest of the ingredients is key to what makes these so light and fluffy.)

3. Stir melted buttery spread into the banana mixture. Stir in sugar, salt, eggs, and vanilla extract.

4. Mix in flour and cinnamon. Stir in walnuts.

5. Scoop batter into prepared muffin tin. Bake for 20 minutes or until a toothpick inserted in the center of a muffin comes out clean. Place muffin tin on a cooling rack and cool for 2 minutes. Remove muffins from tin and place on rack to finish cooling. Store in an airtight container at room temperature for up to 3 days.

Breakfast Cookies

Ingredients :
- 2 large bananas, peeled and mashed
- ¾ cup gluten-free peanut butter
- ¼ cup honey
- 1 tablespoon pure vanilla extract
- 1 tablespoon ground cinnamon
- ¾ teaspoon salt
- ½ cup mini gluten-free and dairy-free chocolate chips
- ½ cup raisins
- 3 cups gluten-free oats

Directions :

1. Preheat oven to 325°F. Line a baking sheet with parchment paper or spray with gluten-free nonstick cooking spray.

2. Add bananas, peanut butter, and honey to a large bowl, and stir to combine. Add vanilla extract, cinnamon, and salt and stir. Stir in the chocolate chips and raisins. Add gluten-free oats. Mix all ingredients together.

3. Use a 1½" tablespoon cookie scoop sprayed with gluten-free nonstick cooking spray to scoop out batter and place onto prepared baking sheet. Flatten the tops slightly. Bake for 15 minutes or until lightly browned. Allow to cool for 2–3 minutes before serving.

Country Breakfast Skillet

Ingredients :
- 2 teaspoons olive oil
- 6 cups frozen cubed hash browns
- ¾ cup seeded and chopped green bell pepper
- ½ cup peeled and chopped sweet onion
- 1 teaspoon salt
- ¼ teaspoon ground black pepper
- 6 large eggs
- 6 cooked gluten-free bacon strips, chopped
- 6 cooked gluten-free sausage links, chopped

Directions :

1. Heat olive oil in a large skillet over medium heat. Add hash browns, bell peppers, onions, salt, and black pepper and cook for 2 minutes, stirring occasionally. Cover and cook for 15 minutes, stirring occasionally, until potatoes are browned and tender.

2. Make six small wells in the potato mixture with a large spoon; break one egg into each well. Cover skillet and cook on low heat for 8–10 minutes or until eggs are completely set. Sprinkle bacon and sausage all over the mixture. Spoon an egg with the potato mixture on each plate and serve warm.

Baked Apple Cinnamon Donuts

Ingredients :

MUFFINS
- ¾ cup sugar
- 2 large eggs
- 1 cup applesauce
- 3 tablespoons vegetable oil
- ½ teaspoon pure vanilla extract
- 1½ cups gluten-free all-purpose flour with xanthan gum
- ½ teaspoon ground cinnamon
- ½ teaspoon salt
- 1 teaspoon gluten-free baking powder

GLAZE
- 1 cup confectioners' sugar
- ¼ teaspoon ground cinnamon
- 1 teaspoon pure vanilla extract
- 4 tablespoons pure maple syrup

Directions :

1. Preheat oven to 350°F. Spray a full-sized sixteen-cup donut pan with gluten-free nonstick cooking spray.

2. In a large bowl, combine sugar, eggs, applesauce, vegetable oil, and vanilla extract. Mix until fully combined.

3. Add flour, cinnamon, salt, and baking powder and mix until fully combined. The batter will be thick and sticky.

4. Add batter to a large plastic storage bag or piping bag. Seal the bag and cut a corner (or tip, if using a piping bag) off. Carefully squeeze batter into donut pan. Bake for 14–16 minutes until golden brown and set. Place plan on a cooling rack and cool for 1 minute. Remove donuts from the pan and place on rack to continue cooling.

5. In a small bowl, whisk together the glaze ingredients. Dip each warm donut into the glaze and place on a plate or wire rack. Store in an airtight container at room temperature for up to 3 days.

Turkey Sausage Patties

Ingredients :
- 1 teaspoon dried thyme
- 1 teaspoon dried sage

- 1 teaspoon onion powder
- ¼ teaspoon garlic powder
- ½ teaspoon salt
- 1 teaspoon pure maple syrup
- 1 pound ground turkey
- 1 tablespoon olive oil

Directions :

1. Combine thyme, sage, onion powder, garlic powder, and salt in a large bowl. Add maple syrup and stir together to combine. Add ground turkey and mix until fully combined.

2. Heat olive oil in a large skillet over medium-high heat.

3. Form turkey sausage into twelve patties and fry 6–8 minutes total until browned on both sides and no longer pink in the center.

Classic French Toast

- **Ingredients :**
- 2 large eggs
- 1 cup unsweetened almond milk
- 1 teaspoon ground cinnamon
- ¼ teaspoon ground nutmeg
- 2 teaspoons pure vanilla extract
- 1 tablespoon granulated sugar
- 8 slices gluten-free and dairy-free bread
- 2 tablespoons dairy-free buttery spread
- ½ cup pure maple syrup

Directions :

1. Whisk together eggs, milk, cinnamon, nutmeg, vanilla extract, and sugar in a pie pan. Place bread slices in the egg mixture and flip to make sure both sides of bread are well coated.

2. Melt buttery spread in a large skillet. Place bread slices in skillet and cook on medium heat for 2–3 minutes on each side until golden brown. Serve warm with maple syrup.

Grilled Chicken Chimichurri Salad

Ingredients :

MARINADE
- 1 cup fresh chopped cilantro
- 1 teaspoon jarred minced garlic
- 2 green onions, sliced

- 1 teaspoon ground cumin
- ½ cup cashew butter
- 4 teaspoons white vinegar
- 1 teaspoon balsamic vinegar
- ½ teaspoon ground turmeric
- ½ cup honey
- ¼ cup olive oil

CHICKEN
- 2 (6-ounce) boneless, skinless chicken breasts
- 2 tablespoons olive oil

SALAD
- 4 cups chopped romaine lettuce
- 2 large avocados, peeled, pitted, and diced
- ¼ cup chopped cilantro
- ½ cup chopped cucumbers
- ¼ cup chopped cashews
- ½ cup halved grape tomatoes
- 2 large hard-boiled eggs, peeled and sliced

Directions :

1. In a food processor, purée cilantro, garlic, green onions, and cumin. In a medium microwave-safe bowl stir together cashew butter, vinegars, turmeric, and honey and microwave for 1 minute. Add the cilantro mixture to the cashew butter mixture and stir until fully combined. Pour olive oil into the combined mixture and stir to finish the marinade. Cover and refrigerate until ready to use.

2. Add chicken breasts and ½ cup of marinade to a sealable plastic bag. Seal the bag and allow chicken to marinate for at least 1 hour.

3. Add olive oil to a grill pan and heat over medium-high heat. Grill chicken for 6–7 minutes on each side until completely cooked (the meat is no longer pink, the juices run clear, and meat reaches an internal temperature of 165°F). Allow chicken to cool for 5 minutes before slicing.

4. Portion salad ingredients on four plates. Top with sliced chicken and drizzle with remaining sauce.

Smoked Salmon Sushi Bowls

Ingredients :

SUSHI RICE
- 2 cups sushi rice
- 2 tablespoons rice vinegar
- 1 tablespoon granulated sugar

- 2 teaspoons salt

SOY GINGER DRESSING
- ½ cup gluten-free soy sauce
- ¼ cup rice vinegar
- 2 tablespoons honey
- 1 teaspoon sesame oil
- 2 tablespoons minced ginger
- ½ teaspoon jarred minced garlic

BOWL TOPPINGS
- 8 ounces smoked salmon, sliced
- 1½ cups peeled and diced English cucumber
- 1 large avocado, peeled, pitted, and diced
- 2 nori sheets, chopped
- ½ teaspoon toasted black sesame seeds, for garnish

Directions :

1. Cook sushi rice according to the package directions.
2. In a small microwave-safe bowl, mix vinegar, sugar, and salt. Heat in the microwave for 30 seconds and stir until sugar and salt are dissolved. Pour the vinegar mixture over the rice, stirring to coat.
3. In a medium bowl, stir together soy sauce, vinegar, honey, sesame oil, ginger, and garlic. Whisk until honey is dissolved.
4. Portion rice into four bowls and top with smoked salmon, cucumber, avocado, and nori. Drizzle the top with the soy ginger dressing. Sprinkle with sesame seeds.

Asian Chicken Lettuce Wraps

Ingredients :
- 1 teaspoon olive oil
- 1 pound ground chicken
- 1½ teaspoons jarred minced garlic
- 1 cup peeled and diced sweet onion
- 2 teaspoons sesame oil
- ¼ cup gluten-free soy sauce
- 1 teaspoon rice wine vinegar
- 1 tablespoon jarred minced ginger
- ¼ teaspoon sriracha
- 1 teaspoon light brown sugar, packed
- 1 tablespoon gluten-free peanut butter

- 1 (8-ounce) can water chestnuts, drained and chopped
- 3 green onions, thinly sliced
- 1 head butter lettuce

Directions :

1. Heat olive oil in a large skillet over medium-high heat. Add ground chicken, garlic, and sweet onions and cook for 5–6 minutes until browned, making sure to crumble the chicken as it cooks. Drain excess grease.

2. In a medium bowl, whisk together sesame oil, soy sauce, vinegar, ginger, sriracha, brown sugar, and peanut butter until fully combined.

3. Add the sauce mixture to chicken and stir to combine. Bring sauce to a low boil. Stir in chestnuts and green onions and cook for 2–3 minutes until tender.

4. To serve, spoon the chicken mixture into the center of lettuce leaves, fold, and enjoy.

Creamy Italian Pasta Salad

Ingredients :

PASTA
- 1 (12-ounce) box gluten-free rotini pasta

CREAMY ITALIAN DRESSING
- 1 teaspoon garlic powder
- 1 teaspoon onion powder
- 1 teaspoon dried basil
- 1 teaspoon dried oregano
- 1 teaspoon dried parsley
- ½ teaspoon dried thyme
- ½ teaspoon dried marjoram
- 1½ teaspoons salt
- ½ teaspoon ground black pepper
- 2 tablespoons granulated sugar
- 1 cup mayonnaise
- 1 tablespoon red wine vinegar
- 1 tablespoon balsamic vinegar

PASTA SALAD
- 1 (14-ounce) can artichoke hearts, drained and chopped
- 1 cup sliced black olives
- 1 cup quartered grape tomatoes
- 1 cup diced roasted red peppers

- ¼ cup chopped fresh basil

Directions :

1. Cook pasta to al dente per the box directions. After draining the pasta, rinse pasta with cold water and allow to cool, then add to a large bowl.

2. In a small bowl, add all the dressing ingredients together and stir until fully combined.

3. Add artichokes, olives, tomatoes, red peppers, and dressing to pasta and stir until fully coated. Cover and refrigerate for 30 minutes before serving. Sprinkle with basil before serving.

Tuna Salad Avocado Bowls

Ingredients :
- ¼ cup mayonnaise
- ½ teaspoon Old Bay Seasoning
- ½ teaspoon dried dill
- 2 tablespoons sweet pickle relish
- ½ teaspoon lemon juice
- 2 large avocados, pitted and halved
- 2 (5-ounce) cans tuna, drained
- 1 large hard-boiled egg, peeled and chopped

Directions :

1. In a large bowl, whisk together mayonnaise, Old Bay Seasoning, dill, relish, and lemon juice.

2. Scoop out some of the avocados from the pitted areas to widen the areas. Place scooped avocado in a small bowl and mash with a fork.

3. Add mashed avocado and tuna to the mayonnaise mixture and stir until well blended. Once fully combined, add egg and stir until well blended. Add tuna salad into the center of each avocado half.

Southern Chicken Salad

Ingredients :
- ¾ cup mayonnaise
- ¼ teaspoon seasoned salt
- 2 tablespoons gluten–free and dairy-free honey mustard salad dressing
- 1 teaspoon lemon juice
- 4 cups chopped, cooked chicken breast
- 1 large Gala apple, peeled, cored, and chopped

Directions :

1. In a large bowl, whisk together mayonnaise, seasoned salt, honey mustard dressing, and lemon juice.

2. Add chicken and stir until well blended, then add apples and stir until well blended.

3. Cover and refrigerate for 30 minutes before serving.

Taco Salad

Ingredients :

TACO MEAT
- 1 teaspoon olive oil
- 1 pound 90/10 ground beef
- 1 tablespoon ground cumin
- 2 teaspoons onion powder
- ½ teaspoon garlic powder
- 2 teaspoons paprika
- 2 teaspoons dried oregano
- ½ teaspoon salt

SALAD
- 1 (15-ounce) can corn, drained
- 1 (15-ounce) can black beans, drained and rinsed
- 1 cup halved grape tomatoes
- 2 large avocados, peeled, pitted, and chopped
- ½ cup sliced black olives
- ½ cup chopped fresh cilantro
- 1 large romaine lettuce heart, chopped
- ½ cup crushed gluten-free tortilla chips

Directions :

1. Heat olive oil in a large skillet over medium-high heat. Add ground beef and seasonings and break up ground beef into equal-sized pieces as it cooks. Cook for 5–8 minutes until browned and broken into crumbles; drain oil.
2. Add salad ingredients except tortilla chips to a large bowl and toss to combine. Top with beef and tortilla chips.

Soy Ginger Vegetable Stir-Fry

Ingredients :
- ¼ cup gluten-free soy sauce
- 2 tablespoons rice vinegar
- 2 tablespoons light brown sugar, packed
- 2 tablespoons cornstarch
- 1 tablespoon jarred minced ginger

- 1 teaspoon sesame oil
- ¼ teaspoon sriracha
- 2 tablespoons vegetable oil
- 1 tablespoon jarred minced garlic
- 2 cups broccoli florets
- 1 cup peeled and sliced carrots
- 1 medium sweet onion, peeled and thinly sliced
- 1 large red bell pepper, seeded and cut into strips
- 1 cup sliced white button mushrooms
- 2 cups sugar snap peas
- 1 teaspoon sesame seeds

Directions :

1. In a small bowl add soy sauce, rice vinegar, brown sugar, cornstarch, ginger, sesame oil, and sriracha and whisk until combined.

2. Heat vegetable oil in a large wok or skillet over medium-high heat. Add garlic, broccoli, carrots, onions, and peppers, and cook for 2–3 minutes. Add mushrooms and snap peas and allow to cook for 2–3 minutes longer.

3. Stir in sauce and allow to cook for 1–2 minutes until vegetables are coated and sauce has thickened.

4. Sprinkle with sesame seeds.

Southwest Tricolored Quinoa Salad

Ingredients :
- 4 tablespoons olive oil
- 1 tablespoon lime juice
- 1 tablespoon honey
- 1 tablespoon ground cumin
- ¼ teaspoon salt
- ½ cup chopped fresh cilantro
- 1 cup tricolored quinoa
- 1 large avocado, peeled, pitted, and diced
- 1 cup canned black beans, drained and rinsed
- 1 cup canned corn, drained
- 1 cup grape tomatoes, quartered

Directions :

1. In a small bowl, whisk together olive oil, lime juice, honey, cumin, and salt until fully combined. Add cilantro and stir.

2. Cook quinoa according to the package directions. Allow to cool.
3. Place cooled quinoa, avocado, beans, corn, and tomatoes in a large bowl. Pour dressing over salad and stir to fully coat and serve. Store leftovers in an airtight container for up to 3 days.

Avocado Bacon Chicken Salad

Ingredients :
- 3 tablespoons lime juice
- 3 tablespoons olive oil
- 1 teaspoon salt
- ¼ teaspoon gluten- and dairy-free hot sauce
- 4 cups chopped cooked chicken breast
- 2 large avocados, peeled, pitted, and diced
- 1 cup chopped cooked gluten-free bacon
- 1 cup canned corn, drained
- ¼ cup chopped fresh cilantro

Directions :
1. In a small bowl whisk together lime juice, olive oil, salt, and pepper sauce until fully combined.
2. In a large bowl add chicken, avocado, bacon, corn, and cilantro and stir to combine.
3. Drizzle dressing over chicken salad and toss to combine. Cover and refrigerate for 30 minutes before serving.

Southwestern Chicken Salad

Ingredients :
- ¼ cup olive oil
- ¼ cup lime juice
- ¼ cup honey
- 2 teaspoons ground cumin
- ½ teaspoon garlic powder
- ¼ teaspoon gluten- and dairy-free hot sauce
- ½ teaspoon salt
- 4 cups chopped cooked chicken breast
- 1 (15-ounce) can corn, drained
- 1 (15-ounce) can black beans, drained and rinsed
- 1 cup chopped roasted red peppers
- 1 cup peeled and chopped red onion
- 1 cup chopped fresh cilantro
- 2 large avocados, peeled, pitted, and chopped

Directions :

1. In a small bowl, whisk together olive oil, lime juice, honey, cumin, garlic powder, pepper sauce, and salt until fully combined.

2. In a large bowl, add chicken, corn, beans, red peppers, onions, cilantro, and avocado.

3. Pour lime sauce over the chicken mixture and toss to coat. Cover and refrigerate for 30 minutes before serving.

Chopped Asian Salad with Peanut Dressing

Ingredients :

PEANUT DRESSING
- 2 tablespoons gluten-free peanut butter
- 1 tablespoon gluten-free soy sauce
- 1 tablespoon sesame oil
- 2 tablespoons water
- 1 tablespoon rice wine vinegar
- 1 tablespoon lime juice
- ½ teaspoon jarred minced garlic
- ½ teaspoon jarred minced ginger
- 1 tablespoon honey
- ½ teaspoon sriracha
- ½ teaspoon salt
- ¼ teaspoon ground black pepper

SALAD
- 1 (14-ounce) package dairy-free coleslaw mix
- 2 carrots, peeled and cut into matchsticks
- 1 cup chopped snow peas
- 1 red bell pepper, seeded and finely diced
- ½ cup fresh chopped cilantro
- ¼ cup chopped green onion
- 1 (11-ounce) can mandarin oranges, drained
- 2 tablespoons sesame seeds
- ½ cup chopped peanuts

Directions :

1. In a small bowl, add peanut butter, soy sauce, sesame oil, water, vinegar, lime juice, garlic, ginger, honey, sriracha, salt, and black pepper. Whisk together until fully combined.

2. In a large bowl, toss coleslaw mix, carrots, snow peas, bell peppers, cilantro, and green onions.

3. Add mandarin oranges, sesame seeds, and peanuts to the top of the salad and drizzle with peanut dressing.

Egg Roll Bowl

Ingredients :
- 1 tablespoon sesame oil
- 1 pound ground pork
- 1 tablespoon jarred minced garlic
- 1 sweet onion, peeled and diced
- ½ cup sliced white button mushrooms
- ½ cup gluten-free chicken broth
- 1 tablespoon minced ginger
- ¼ cup gluten-free soy sauce
- 1 tablespoon rice wine vinegar
- 1 (14-ounce) bag dairy-free coleslaw mix

Directions :

1. In a wok or large skillet, heat oil over medium heat. Add ground pork, garlic, onions, and mushrooms and cook for 6–8 minutes until pork is no longer pink and vegetables are tender.

2. In a small bowl, whisk together broth, ginger, soy sauce, and vinegar until fully combined.

3. Pour sauce in skillet and stir in coleslaw mix. Cover and simmer for 5–10 minutes until cabbage is wilted.

Homestyle Egg Salad

Ingredients :
- 6 tablespoons mayonnaise
- 2 teaspoons Dijon mustard
- 1 tablespoon dried dill
- 2 tablespoons dill pickle relish
- ½ teaspoon salt
- ¼ teaspoon ground black pepper
- ¼ cup chopped celery
- 12 large hard-boiled eggs, peeled and chopped

Directions :

1. In a large bowl, combine mayonnaise, mustard, dill, relish, salt, and pepper and stir to combine.

2. Add celery and eggs and stir to combines. Cover and chill for at least 1 hour before serving.

Greek Chicken Wraps

Ingredients :

CHICKEN MARINADE
- ¼ cup olive oil
- ¼ cup red wine vinegar
- ½ cup lemon juice
- 2 teaspoons jarred minced garlic
- 1 teaspoon onion powder
- 1 tablespoon dried oregano
- 2 teaspoons dried thyme
- 1 teaspoon salt
- 1 teaspoon ground black pepper
- 2 (6-ounce) boneless, skinless chicken breasts, sliced into 1" pieces

CUCUMBER SAUCE
- ½ cup peeled and finely diced English cucumber
- 2 tablespoons lemon juice
- 1 tablespoon jarred minced garlic
- 2 tablespoons dried dill
- 1 cup mayonnaise
- ¼ teaspoon salt

CHICKEN WRAP
- 2 tablespoons olive oil
- 4 pieces warm gluten-free Flatbread
- ½ cup diced tomatoes

Directions :

1. In a gallon-sized sealable plastic bag, add olive oil, vinegar, lemon juice, garlic, onion powder, oregano, thyme, salt, and pepper. Add chicken, seal bag, and massage ingredients to combine. Let chicken marinate in the refrigerator for 30 minutes.

2. While chicken is marinating, combine the cucumber sauce ingredients in a small bowl. Cover and refrigerate.

3. Heat olive oil in a large skillet over medium heat. Pour chicken and marinade into the skillet. Stir and cook chicken for 6–7 minutes until it is no longer pink and is fully cooked.

4. Serve over Flatbread pieces. Sprinkle with diced tomatoes and drizzle with cucumber sauce.

Mediterranean Tuna Salad

- **Ingredients :**
- 2 tablespoons olive oil
- 1 tablespoon balsamic vinegar
- 1 teaspoon dried basil
- ½ teaspoon onion powder
- ½ teaspoon salt
- 2 (5-ounce) cans tuna in water, drained
- 1 (15-ounce) can cannellini beans, drained
- 1 cucumber, diced
- 2 large beefsteak tomatoes, diced
- 2 tablespoons chopped Kalamata olives

Directions :

1. In a small bowl, whisk together olive oil, vinegar, basil, onion powder, and salt until fully combined.
2. In a large bowl, combine tuna, beans, cucumbers, tomatoes, and olives. Pour dressing over the tuna mixture and stir to fully combine. Refrigerate for 30 minutes before serving.

Mini Corn Dog Bites

Ingredients :
- 1 box gluten-free corn bread mix with necessary gluten-free and dairy-free ingredients
- 6 gluten-free and dairy-free hot dogs

Directions :

1. Preheat oven according to corn bread mix package directions. Spray twenty-four-cup mini muffin tin with gluten-free nonstick cooking spray.
2. Make corn bread according to the package directions. Fill muffin tin with batter.
3. Cut hot dogs into bite-sized pieces. Place hot dog pieces in the center of each cup filled with batter.
4. Bake according to the package directions.

Spinach Salad with Warm Bacon Dressing

Ingredients :
- 1 teaspoon olive oil
- 8 strips gluten-free bacon
- 1 small red onion, peeled and thinly sliced
- 2 cups sliced white button mushrooms
- 3 tablespoons red wine vinegar
- 2 teaspoons honey
- ½ teaspoon Dijon mustard

- ½ teaspoon salt
- 1 (8-ounce) package baby spinach
- 4 large hard-boiled eggs, peeled and sliced

Directions :

1. Heat olive oil in a large skillet over medium-high heat. Add bacon and fry for 3–4 minutes on each side until brown and crispy. Remove cooked bacon to a paper towel to drain. Once cooled, crumble and set aside. Transfer 3 tablespoons bacon grease from the skillet to a small saucepan. Safely disregard the remaining oil.

2. Add onions and mushrooms to the skillet and cook on medium heat for 3–5 minutes until onions and mushrooms are caramelized and reduced.

3. Add vinegar, honey, mustard, and salt into saucepan with bacon grease. Whisk together and heat thoroughly for 2 minutes over medium-low heat.

4. Add spinach to a large bowl. Top with sautéed onions, mushrooms, and bacon. Pour hot dressing over salad and toss to combine. Place sliced eggs on top and serve.

Crispy Southwest Wraps

Ingredients :
- 1 pound 90/10 ground beef
- ½ large red bell pepper, seeded and chopped
- ½ teaspoon salt
- ⅛ teaspoon ground black pepper
- 2 teaspoons chili powder
- 2 teaspoons ground cumin
- 2 teaspoons garlic powder
- 2 teaspoons onion powder
- 1 teaspoon dried oregano
- 3 tablespoons water
- 1 (15-ounce) can black beans, drained and rinsed
- 1 cup canned corn, drained
- ½ cup chopped fresh cilantro
- 6 large gluten-free and dairy-free flour tortillas
- 1 cup cooked rice
- 3 tablespoons vegetable oil

Directions :

1. Add beef to a large skillet and cook for 5–8 minutes over medium heat until crumbled and browned; drain grease.

2. Add bell peppers to the skillet and cook for 2 minutes until tender. Add salt, pepper, chili powder, cumin, garlic powder, onion powder, oregano, and water. Stir to combine. Add black beans, corn, and cilantro and stir to combine. Cook for 2–3 minutes.

3. Heat each tortilla in the microwave for 10 seconds to make it easier to roll. Add rice to the center of each tortilla and top with the beef mixture. Roll up, folding in the sides like a burrito.

4. Spray a large skillet with gluten-free nonstick cooking spray and place the wraps seam-side down.

5. Gently brush the tops of the wraps lightly with oil. Cook for 2 minutes on each side on medium-high heat until golden and crispy.

Loaded Burger Bowls

Ingredients :

BURGERS
- 1 pound 90/10 ground beef
- 1 teaspoon seasoned salt
- 1 teaspoon olive oil
- 8 strips gluten-free bacon, chopped
- ½ cup peeled and thinly sliced sweet onion
- ½ cup sliced white button mushrooms

SPECIAL SAUCE
- ½ cup mayonnaise
- 3 tablespoons ketchup
- 2 tablespoons sweet pickle relish
- 1½ teaspoons granulated sugar
- 1½ teaspoons white vinegar
- ¼ teaspoon onion powder
- ¼ teaspoon salt

BOWLS
- 1 head iceberg lettuce, chopped
- 1 cup halved grape tomatoes
- ½ cup chopped dill pickles

Directions :

1. In a medium bowl, mix together beef and seasoned salt.

2. Heat olive oil in a large skillet over medium heat, then add bacon and cook for 2–3 minutes on each side until brown and crispy. Remove to a paper towel–lined plate to drain.

3. Add beef to the skillet and cook for 4–6 minutes until starting to brown and crumble. Stir in onions

and mushrooms and cook for 2–3 minutes until onions and mushrooms have started to caramelize and get soft.

4. In a small bowl, whisk together the sauce ingredients until fully combined.

5. To assemble bowls, start with a layer of chopped lettuce, then spoon the beef mixture into the center. Arrange tomatoes, pickles, and bacon around the beef and drizzle with sauce and serve.

Grilled Chicken Caesar Salad

Ingredients :

CHICKEN
- 2 (6-ounce) boneless, skinless chicken breasts
- 2 tablespoons olive oil, divided
- 2 tablespoons lemon juice
- ½ teaspoon salt
- ¼ teaspoon ground black pepper
- 1 teaspoon jarred minced garlic

CAESAR DRESSING
- ½ cup mayonnaise
- 1 teaspoon gluten-free Worcestershire sauce
- 1 tablespoon lemon juice
- 2 teaspoons jarred minced garlic
- 1 teaspoon Dijon mustard
- 1 teaspoon olive oil
- ¼ teaspoon salt
- ⅛ teaspoon ground black pepper

CROUTONS
- ½ cup olive oil
- 1 teaspoon garlic powder
- 1 teaspoon onion powder
- ¼ teaspoon salt
- 4 cups cubed gluten-free and dairy-free bread

SALAD
- 4 large romaine lettuce hearts, chopped

Directions :

1. Place chicken in a sealable plastic bag. Add 1 tablespoon oil, lemon juice, salt, pepper, and garlic. Seal the top of the bag and massage the ingredients to combine. Let chicken marinate for 30 minutes.

2. In a small bowl, whisk together the Caesar dressing ingredients until combined. Cover and refrigerate.

3. Preheat oven to 375°F. Line a baking sheet with parchment paper.

4. In a small bowl, whisk together olive oil, garlic powder, onion powder, and salt. In a large bowl, add bread, drizzle with the olive oil mixture, and toss. Spread bread in one even layer on prepared baking sheet. Bake for 10 minutes. Remove the pan from oven, toss cubes, and return to the oven. Bake for 5 minutes until crisp and golden brown.

5. Heat remaining 1 tablespoon oil on a grill pan over medium-high heat. Grill chicken for 7 minutes per side until completely cooked; the meat should reach an internal temperature of 165°F. Allow chicken to cool before slicing it for the salad.

6. Add dressing to a large bowl, add lettuce, and toss. Add sliced grilled chicken and croutons on top of lettuce and serve.

Grilled Chicken Cobb Salad

- **Ingredients :**
- 2 (6-ounce) boneless, skinless chicken breasts
- 2 tablespoons olive oil, divided
- 2 tablespoons lemon juice
- 1 teaspoon jarred minced garlic
- ½ teaspoon salt
- ¼ teaspoon ground black pepper
- 3 medium romaine lettuce hearts, chopped
- 8 strips gluten-free bacon, cooked and crumbled
- 1 cup canned corn, drained
- 4 large hard-boiled eggs, peeled and chopped
- 1 cup halved grape tomatoes
- 2 large avocados, peeled, pitted, and chopped

Directions :

1. Place chicken breasts in a sealable plastic bag. Add 1 tablespoon olive oil, lemon juice, garlic, salt, and pepper. Seal the top of the bag and massage the ingredients to combine. Let chicken marinate in the refrigerator for 30 minutes.

2. Heat remaining olive oil in a large skillet over medium-high heat. Grill chicken for 6–7minutes on each side until completely cooked; the meat should no longer be pink, the juices should run clear, and it should reach an internal temperature of 165°F. Allow chicken to cool for 5 minutes before slicing it for the salad.

3. In a large bowl, add lettuce and top with chicken, bacon, corn, eggs, tomatoes, and avocado.

Broiled Romaine Salad with Balsamic Glaze

Ingredients :

GLAZE
- 2 teaspoons balsamic vinegar
- 2 tablespoons honey
- 2 tablespoons olive oil
- 1 teaspoon garlic powder
- ½ teaspoon onion powder
- ¼ teaspoon Dijon mustard
- ¼ teaspoon salt
- ⅛ teaspoon ground black pepper

ROMAINE
- 1 large romaine lettuce heart, halved
- ½ tablespoon olive oil

Directions :

1. In a small bowl, whisk together the glaze ingredients until fully combined. Microwave for 15 seconds and then whisk again. Allow to cool before drizzling on romaine.

2. Place romaine on a baking sheet sprayed with gluten-free nonstick cooking spray. Drizzle the lettuce with the olive oil and place under the broiler for 1–2 minutes. Flip when the leaves start to brown a bit, then cook for 1–2 minutes more.

3. Remove from oven, plate, and drizzle with balsamic glaze.

Sloppy Joe Baked Potatoes

Ingredients :
- 4 large russet potatoes
- 1 teaspoon olive oil
- 1 pound 90/10 ground beef
- ¼ teaspoon salt
- 1 (15-ounce) can gluten-free Sloppy Joe sauce

Directions :

1. With a fork, pierce each potato several times. Wrap each potato in microwaveable plastic wrap and place on a microwave-safe plate. Microwave on high for 6 minutes; turn over and microwave for an additional 5 minutes until soft. Remove and allow to cool for 5 minutes.

2. Heat olive oil in a large skillet over medium-high heat. Add beef and salt, stirring occasionally, and cook for 5 minutes until crumbled and no longer pink; then drain the oil. Add sauce. Reduce heat to

low and simmer 5 minutes until hot.

3. Cut slit in top of each potato; squeeze open and fluff with fork. Top each potato with ½ cup meat mixture.

Traditional Greek Salad

Ingredients :
- 1 romaine lettuce heart, chopped
- 1 large cucumber, sliced
- 1 green bell pepper, seeded and diced
- 1 pint grape tomatoes, halved
- ½ small red onion, peeled and thinly sliced
- 1 teaspoon jarred minced garlic
- 1 teaspoon dried oregano
- ½ teaspoon Dijon mustard
- ¼ cup red wine vinegar
- 1 teaspoon salt
- ½ teaspoon ground black pepper
- ½ cup olive oil
- ½ cup halved pitted Kalamata olives

Directions :

1. Add lettuce, cucumber, bell peppers, tomatoes, and red onions in a large bowl.

2. In a small bowl, whisk together garlic, oregano, mustard, vinegar, salt, and pepper. Whisk in olive oil. Pour vinaigrette over vegetables. Add olives and toss lightly.

Spinach and Artichoke Chicken

Ingredients :
- 4 tablespoons olive oil
- 4 (6-ounce) boneless, skinless chicken breasts
- 2 tablespoons jarred minced garlic
- 1 small sweet onion, peeled and chopped
- 1 cup gluten-free chicken broth
- 1 tablespoon gluten-free Worcestershire sauce
- 1 tablespoon lemon juice
- 1 teaspoon salt
- 1 cup unsweetened almond milk
- 2 tablespoons gluten-free all-purpose flour with xanthan gum
- 4 tablespoons nutritional yeast
- 1 (6-ounce) bag baby spinach

- 1 (13-ounce) can artichoke hearts

Directions :

1. Heat olive oil in a large skillet over medium-high heat. Add chicken and cook for 2 minutes on each side. Remove chicken to a plate.

2. Add garlic and onions to the skillet and stir, cooking for 30 seconds, until garlic is fragrant. Pour in broth, Worcestershire sauce, lemon juice, and salt and stir to combine. Add chicken back into the skillet and turn down the heat to medium and cook for 12–14 minutes, turning over the chicken about halfway through.

3. Transfer chicken to a plate. Combine milk, flour, and nutritional yeast in a small bowl and whisk until flour is dissolved. Pour the mixture into the skillet, stir, and bring to a low boil.

4. Add spinach to sauce and cover and cook for 2–3 minutes until wilted. Stir in artichoke hearts and cook for 2–3 minutes until heated through. Pour creamy sauce over chicken and serve.

Crispy Baked Barbecue Chicken Thighs

- **Ingredients :**
- 1 tablespoon light brown sugar, packed
- 1 tablespoon garlic powder
- 1 tablespoon onion powder
- 1 tablespoon chili powder
- 1 tablespoon salt
- 1 tablespoon paprika
- 1 tablespoon ground cumin
- 1 teaspoon mustard powder
- 6 (4-ounce) bone-in, skin-on chicken thighs
- ¾ cup gluten-free bread crumbs
- ½ cup dairy-free buttery spread

Directions :

1. Preheat oven to 375°F. Spray a 9" × 13" glass baking dish with gluten-free nonstick cooking spray. Place chicken in baking dish.

2. In a small bowl, combine brown sugar, garlic powder, onion powder, chili powder, salt, paprika, cumin, and mustard powder together and stir until fully combined.

3. Rub 1 tablespoon seasoning mixture on each chicken thigh.

4. Sprinkle bread crumbs over chicken thighs and press onto skin.

5. Drizzle buttery spread over chicken thighs.

6. Bake for 50 minutes or until the thighs are no longer pink at the bone and the juices run clear. A meat thermometer inserted near the bone should read 165°F.

Paleo Pesto Turkey Meatballs

Ingredients :

PESTO SAUCE
- 1 (10-ounce) package fresh basil
- 1 cup cashews
- 2 tablespoons jarred minced garlic
- 1 teaspoon salt
- 2 tablespoons lemon juice
- ½ cup olive oil

MEATBALLS
- 3 pounds ground turkey
- 2 large eggs, whisked
- ⅔ cup almond flour
- 2 tablespoons onion powder

Directions :

1. Preheat oven to 425°F. Line two baking sheets with aluminum foil and spray with gluten-free nonstick cooking spray.

2. In a food processor, chop the basil. Add cashews to the food processor and chop until fully combined with basil. Add the garlic, salt, lemon juice and olive oil to the cashew mixture and chop until fully combined.

3. To make the meatballs, add turkey, eggs, almond flour, onion powder, and pesto sauce to a large bowl. Mix together with a large spoon or your hands until fully combined.

4. Using a 1½-tablespoons cookie scoop, scoop the meatball mixture out to form forty-eight balls and place on prepared baking sheets. Bake for 30 minutes until browned.

Crunchy Coconut Chicken Bites

Ingredients :
- 2 cups Honey Nut Chex cereal
- 1 cup sweetened shredded coconut
- 2 boneless, skinless chicken breasts, cut into 2" pieces
- ½ cup mayonnaise
- ½ cup orange marmalade, melted

Directions :

1. Preheat oven to 400°F. Line a baking sheet with aluminum foil and spray with gluten-free nonstick cooking spray.

2. Crush cereal by adding it to a sealable plastic bag and crushing with a rolling pin. Add coconut to the bag.

3. Combine chicken and mayonnaise in a medium bowl and transfer to the bag with the cereal mixture. Turn the plastic storage bag over and over until the chicken pieces are coated evenly.

4. Place chicken on prepared baking sheet and bake for 18–20 minutes until the coating is a light golden brown. Serve with melted orange marmalade as a dipping sauce.

Turmeric Coconut Chicken Curry

Ingredients :
- 1 tablespoon olive oil
- 2 (6-ounce) boneless, skinless chicken breasts, cut into 1" pieces
- 1 (13-ounce) can unsweetened coconut milk
- 2 tablespoons honey
- 1 teaspoon ground cinnamon
- 1 teaspoon ground turmeric
- ½ teaspoon ground ginger
- ¼ teaspoon salt
- ½ cup raisins
- 2 large hard-boiled eggs, peeled and diced
- ½ cup chopped fresh cilantro

Directions :

1. Heat the olive oil in a large skillet over medium-high heat. Sauté chicken for 5–6 minutes until golden brown.

2. Add milk and honey and stir, coating chicken. Add spices and raisins and stir to combine ingredients.

3. Bring to a low boil, then lower heat to low and simmer for 5 minutes, stirring occasionally, until sauce thickens.

4. Plate chicken and garnish with hard-boiled eggs and cilantro.

Asian Apricot Chicken

Ingredients :

CHICKEN
- ½ cup gluten-free all-purpose flour with xanthan gum
- ½ cup gluten-free cornstarch

- 1 tablespoon ground ginger
- 2 (6-ounce) boneless, skinless chicken breasts, cut into 1" pieces
- 1 large egg, whisked
- 2 cups vegetable oil

SAUCE
- 2 tablespoons gluten-free soy sauce
- 1 teaspoon ground ginger
- ¾ cup apricot preserves
- ¼ cup water

Directions :

1. Combine flour, cornstarch, and ground ginger in a large sealable plastic bag.

2. Add chicken pieces to a medium bowl with whisked egg and stir to fully coat the pieces.

3. Place all chicken pieces in the bag of flour mixture. Keep turning over the bag until chicken pieces are fully coated.

4. Heat oil in a wok or large skillet over high heat until a deep-fry thermometer inserted in the oil registers 350°F. Carefully add chicken and fry for 3–4 minutes, turning once or twice, until golden brown and crisp. Drain the chicken on a paper towel–lined plate. Carefully pour hot oil from pan into a bowl and dispose of safely once cooled.

5. Either spray your pan with a gluten-free nonstick cooking spray or put 1 teaspoon fresh oil back into wok. Add all the sauce ingredients. Stir until combined, then cook over medium heat for 1–2 minutes until sauce thickens.

6. Return fried chicken to the pan, cook for 2–3 minutes more, and stir to evenly coat chicken with the sauce.

Oven-Fried Chicken

Ingredients :
- 1 cup unsweetened almond milk
- 1 tablespoon white vinegar
- 4 pounds chicken pieces (thighs, breasts, wings, and drum sticks)
- 1 cup gluten-free all-purpose flour with xanthan gum
- 1 cup gluten-free bread crumbs
- 1 tablespoon seasoned salt
- 1 tablespoon dried thyme
- 1 tablespoon onion powder
- 1 teaspoon garlic powder
- 1 teaspoon dried basil
- 1 teaspoon dried oregano

- ½ teaspoon mustard powder

Directions :

1. Pour milk and vinegar in a small bowl and allow to sit for 5 minutes. Pour the mixture in a sealable plastic bag and then place chicken into the bag and seal. Massage chicken and the milk mixture with your hands to coat evenly and allow to marinate in the refrigerator for 30 minutes up to several hours.

2. Preheat oven to 375°F and spray a 9" × 13" baking dish with gluten-free nonstick cooking spray.

3. In a medium bowl, whisk together flour, bread crumbs, and seasonings. Set aside.

4. Remove chicken from the bag and dredge in the seasoned flour mixture, coating on all sides. Place chicken into prepared baking dish. Spray the tops of chicken pieces with gluten-free nonstick cooking spray. Bake for 50 minutes until internal temperature reads 165°F. Remove from oven and allow to rest 5 minutes and serve.

Chicken and Dumplings Casserole

Ingredients :
- ½ cup dairy-free buttery spread, melted
- 4 (6-ounce) boneless, skinless chicken breasts, cooked and shredded
- ½ teaspoon salt
- ½ teaspoon ground black pepper
- 1 teaspoon dried sage
- ½ cup frozen peas
- ½ cup frozen corn
- 2 cups unsweetened almond milk
- 2 cups Bisquick Gluten Free Pancake & Baking Mix
- 1 cup gluten-free chicken broth
- 3 teaspoons gluten-free chicken granules
- 1½ cups gluten-free and dairy-free Cream of Chicken Soup

Directions :

1. Preheat oven to 350°F. Spray a 9" × 13" baking dish with gluten-free nonstick cooking spray.

2. Pour buttery spread into bottom of baking dish. Spread chicken over buttery spread. Sprinkle salt, pepper, and sage over chicken. Sprinkle peas and corn over chicken. Do not stir.

3. To make the second layer, mix milk and Bisquick in a small bowl. Pour the mixture on top of peas and corn. Do not stir.

4. To make the third layer, whisk together broth, chicken granules, and soup. Once blended, slowly pour over the Bisquick layer. Do not stir.

5. Bake casserole for 45–60 minutes or until the top is golden brown.

Moroccan Chicken

Ingredients :
- 3 tablespoons olive oil
- ¼ teaspoon salt
- ⅛ teaspoon ground black pepper
- 6 (4-ounce) skin-on chicken thighs
- 1 large sweet onion, peeled and chopped
- 2 tablespoons jarred minced garlic
- 1 tablespoon ground turmeric
- 1 tablespoon ground cumin
- 1 teaspoon ground cinnamon
- 1 teaspoon paprika
- 2 teaspoons lemon zest
- 1 tablespoon lemon juice
- 3 cups gluten-free chicken broth
- 4 tablespoons honey
- 1 tablespoon gluten-free all-purpose flour with xanthan gum
- ½ cup raisins
- 2 (10-ounce) packages frozen garbanzos and lentils
- ½ cup chopped fresh cilantro

Directions :

1. Heat olive oil in a large skillet on medium-high.
2. Salt and pepper both sides of chicken.
3. Cook chicken for 6–7 minutes on each side until they are crispy. Remove and transfer to plate.
4. Add onions and garlic to the skillet and sauté in remaining oil for 5 minutes. Add turmeric, cumin, cinnamon, paprika, lemon zest, and lemon juice and stir until fully combined. Add broth, honey, and flour and stir until flour is dissolved.
5. Return chicken to the skillet, cover, and simmer for 15 minutes.
6. Remove lid and add raisins and packages of garbanzos and lentils. Stir to combine in sauce. Cook for an additional 15–20 minutes uncovered.
7. Sprinkle with cilantro to garnish.

Chicken Alfredo

Ingredients :
- 1 (16-ounce) box gluten-free fettuccine
- 2 tablespoons olive oil, divided

- 2 (6-ounce) boneless, skinless chicken breasts
- ¾ teaspoon salt, divided
- ¼ teaspoon ground black pepper
- 4 tablespoons dairy-free buttery spread
- 1 tablespoon jarred minced garlic
- 1 tablespoon onion powder
- 1 cup gluten-free chicken broth
- ½ teaspoon dry mustard powder
- 2 cups unsweetened almond milk
- 4 tablespoons gluten-free all-purpose flour with xanthan gum
- ½ cup nutritional yeast
- ⅛ teaspoon ground nutmeg

Directions :

1. Cook pasta according to package directions until al dente and toss with 1 tablespoon of olive oil.
2. In a large skillet, heat remaining olive oil over medium-high heat. Add chicken and season with ½ teaspoon salt and pepper. Cook chicken until golden and cooked through, 6–7 minutes per side. Remove from the skillet and let rest 10 minutes before slicing.
3. Add buttery spread and garlic to the skillet and sauté for 30 seconds until garlic is fragrant.
4. Add onion powder, chicken broth, mustard powder, and remaining salt and stir until combined.
5. In a small bowl, whisk together milk, flour, and nutritional yeast.
6. Pour the milk mixture into the skillet and stir until fully combined. Reduce heat to medium. Bring to a low boil and stir until sauce is thickened. Sprinkle in nutmeg and stir. Add cooked pasta and toss well to coat pasta with sauce.

Chicken Piccata

Ingredients :
- ½ cup gluten-free all-purpose flour with xanthan gum
- ¼ cup gluten-free cornstarch
- ½ teaspoon salt
- ¼ teaspoon ground black pepper
- 3 (6-ounce) boneless, skinless chicken breasts, cut into ½" medallions
- 2 tablespoons olive oil
- 1 teaspoon jarred minced garlic
- 1 cup gluten-free chicken broth
- ¼ cup lemon juice
- 2 tablespoons capers, drained and rinsed
- 2 tablespoons dairy-free buttery spread

Directions :

1. Preheat oven to 200°F. Line a baking sheet with aluminum foil.

2. Add flour, cornstarch, salt, and pepper to a pie pan and whisk to combine. Dredge chicken pieces in the mixture. Heat olive oil in a large skillet. Pan-fry chicken over medium-high heat for 3 minutes on each side until golden brown. Place chicken pieces on prepared baking sheet and place in the oven to keep warm. Drain most of the oil from the skillet, reserving 1 tablespoon of oil in the skillet.

3. Add garlic to the skillet and cook for 30 seconds until fragrant. Pour in broth. Scrape and dissolve any brown bits from the bottom of the skillet. Stir in lemon juice and bring the mixture to a boil. Boil for 5–8 minutes, stirring occasionally, until the sauce reduces. Add capers and buttery spread and stir to combine until buttery spread is melted.

4. Add chicken back to the skillet and simmer for 5 more minutes until sauce is reduced and slightly thickens. Serve warm.

Tuscan Chicken

Ingredients :
- 2 tablespoons olive oil
- 4 (6-ounce) boneless, skinless chicken breasts
- 2 tablespoons jarred minced garlic
- 1 cup sliced white button mushrooms
- 1 cup gluten-free chicken broth
- 1 tablespoon Italian seasoning
- ½ teaspoon salt
- 4 tablespoons nutritional yeast
- 1 cup unsweetened almond milk
- 2 tablespoons gluten-free all-purpose flour with xanthan gum
- 1 cup chopped baby spinach
- ½ cup chopped sun-dried tomatoes

Directions :

1. In a large skillet, add olive oil and cook chicken on medium-high heat for 3–5 minutes on each side until brown on each side. Remove chicken and set aside on a plate.

2. Add garlic and mushrooms to the skillet and sauté for 2 minutes until mushrooms start to soften.

3. Add chicken broth, Italian seasoning, salt, and nutritional yeast and whisk together.

4. Add milk and flour to a small bowl and whisk until flour has dissolved. Add the milk mixture to the skillet and whisk until it starts to thicken, about 2 minutes.

5. Add spinach and tomatoes to the skillet and let simmer for 2–4 minutes until spinach starts to wilt. Add chicken back to the skillet and simmer for 4–5 minutes.

Crispy Baked Chicken Thighs

- **Ingredients :**
- 6 (4-ounce) bone-in, skin-on chicken thighs
- 1 teaspoon garlic powder
- 1 tablespoon onion powder
- 1 tablespoon dried oregano
- 1 tablespoon dried thyme
- 1 tablespoon dried sage
- 1 teaspoon salt

Directions :

1. Preheat oven to 350°F. Spray a 9" × 13" glass baking pan with gluten-free nonstick cooking spray.

2. Place chicken thighs in greased baking pan.

3. In a small bowl, combine garlic powder, onion powder, oregano, thyme, sage, and salt together and stir until fully combined. Sprinkle the spice mixture over chicken thighs.

4. Bake chicken for 1 hour until skin is crispy, thighs are no longer pink at the bone, and the juices run clear. A meat thermometer inserted near the bone should read 165°F.

Rosemary Roasted Chicken

- **Ingredients :**
- 1 large lemon, halved
- 1 (3-pound) whole chicken, rinsed and patted dry
- 1 tablespoon salt
- 1 teaspoon ground black pepper
- 1 small sweet onion, peeled and quartered
- ¼ cup chopped fresh rosemary

Directions :

1. Preheat oven to 350°F. Spray a medium roasting pan with a rack with gluten-free nonstick cooking spray.

2. Squeeze lemon juice directly over chicken skin. Season chicken with salt and pepper and stuff the inside of chicken with onion, rosemary, and lemon halves. Place chicken with breast-side up on a rack in prepared roasting pan.

3. Roast for 2 to 2½ hours until cooked through, the juices run clear, and internal temperature reaches 165°F.

Honey Garlic Chicken

Ingredients :
- 3 (6-ounce) boneless, skinless chicken breasts, cut into 1" pieces
- ¼ cup gluten-free all-purpose flour with xanthan gum
- ¼ cup gluten-free cornstarch
- ½ teaspoon salt
- ¼ teaspoon ground black pepper
- 4 tablespoons olive oil
- 1 teaspoon jarred minced garlic
- ⅓ cup honey
- 1 tablespoon gluten-free soy sauce
- 1½ tablespoons rice vinegar

Directions :
1. Put chicken pieces in a large sealable plastic bag. Add flour, cornstarch, salt, and pepper to the bag and shake to coat the chicken.
2. Heat oil in a large skillet over medium-high heat and add garlic and sauté for 30 seconds. Add chicken and cook for 3 minutes per side.
3. In a small microwave-safe bowl, whisk together honey, soy sauce, and vinegar and microwave for 15 seconds.
4. Turn heat down to medium. Add honey sauce to the skillet and stir to coat chicken with sauce. Cook for 3–4 minutes more, then serve.

Chicken Scaloppine

Ingredients :
- 4 (6-ounce) boneless, skinless chicken breasts
- 1 tablespoon lemon juice
- ¼ teaspoon salt
- ¼ teaspoon ground black pepper
- ½ cup gluten-free bread crumbs
- 1 teaspoon garlic powder
- 1 teaspoon onion powder
- 1 tablespoon Italian seasoning
- 2 tablespoons olive oil
- ½ cup gluten-free chicken broth
- ¼ cup white wine
- 2 tablespoons capers
- 1 tablespoon dairy-free buttery spread

Directions :
1. Place each chicken breast between two sheets of heavy-duty plastic wrap; pound to ¼" thickness

using a meat mallet or rolling pin. Brush chicken with lemon juice and sprinkle with salt and pepper.

2. In a pie pan, add bread crumbs, garlic powder, onion powder, and Italian seasoning and whisk to combine. Dredge chicken in the bread crumb mixture.

3. In a large skillet, heat olive oil over medium-high heat. Add chicken to pan; cook 3 minutes on each side until chicken is cooked through. Remove chicken from the skillet and cover with aluminum foil to keep warm.

4. Add chicken broth and wine to the skillet and cook for 30 seconds, stirring constantly. Stir in capers and buttery spread.

5. Add chicken back into the skillet, cover with sauce and simmer for 2–4 minutes.

Baked Balsamic Chicken

Ingredients :
- 4 (6-ounce) boneless, skinless chicken breasts
- 1 teaspoon salt, divided
- ¼ teaspoon ground black pepper
- 1 teaspoon Italian seasoning
- 2 tablespoons olive oil
- 1 cup balsamic vinegar
- ½ cup granulated sugar
- 2 tablespoons honey

Directions :

1. Preheat oven to 400°F and spray a 9" × 13" baking dish with gluten-free nonstick cooking spray.

2. Season chicken with ½ teaspoon salt, pepper, and Italian seasoning.

3. Add olive oil to a large skillet and cook chicken on medium-high heat for 2 minutes on each side.

4. Transfer chicken to prepared dish, cover with aluminum foil, and bake for 15 minutes.

5. While chicken is baking, add balsamic vinegar, sugar, honey, and remaining salt to a medium saucepan. Bring to a boil over medium-high heat, then reduce to medium-low heat and allow to simmer 10–15 minutes. The sauce should reduce by half. Remove from heat.

6. Uncover chicken and brush balsamic glaze on top of chicken. Return chicken to the oven and bake uncovered for another 5–10 minutes until chicken is completely cooked through and reaches an internal temperature of 165°F. Drizzle remaining balsamic glaze over chicken and serve.

Sesame Chicken

Ingredients :
- ½ cup gluten-free all-purpose flour with xanthan gum

- ½ cup gluten-free cornstarch
- 2 (6-ounce) boneless, skinless chicken breasts, diced into ½" pieces
- 1 large egg, whisked
- 2 cups vegetable oil
- ¼ cup honey
- ⅓ cup gluten-free soy sauce
- ½ cup ketchup
- ¼ cup light brown sugar, packed
- ¼ cup rice vinegar
- 1 teaspoon jarred minced ginger
- 2 teaspoons cornstarch
- 1 tablespoon sesame oil
- 2 teaspoons jarred minced garlic
- 2 tablespoons sesame seeds
- 2 green onions, sliced

Directions :

1. Combine flour and cornstarch in a large sealable plastic bag. Add chicken to a medium bowl with egg and stir to fully coat pieces. Place chicken in the bag with the flour mixture. Keep turning over the bag until chicken pieces are fully coated.

2. Heat vegetable oil in a large skillet or wok over medium-high heat. Add chicken to hot oil and fry for 6–8 minutes until light golden brown. Drain chicken on a paper towel–lined plate. Discard oil from wok. Allow oil to completely cool before disposing of it.

3. In a small bowl, whisk together honey, soy sauce, ketchup, sugar, vinegar, ginger, and cornstarch until fully combined.

4. Heat sesame oil in the same skillet or wok over medium heat. Add garlic and cook for 30 seconds. Add sauce and bring to a simmer. Cook for 3–4 minutes or until just thickened. Add chicken to the skillet and toss to coat with sauce and cook for 1–2 minutes. Sprinkle with sesame seeds and green onions and serve.

Savory Roasted Milk Chicken Thighs

Ingredients :
- 6 (4-ounce) bone-in, skin-on chicken thighs
- 1 teaspoon ground cumin
- 1 teaspoon paprika
- ½ teaspoon salt
- ¼ teaspoon ground black pepper
- 4 tablespoons dairy-free buttery spread, divided
- 1½ teaspoons jarred minced garlic

- 1 cup unsweetened almond milk
- ¾ cup gluten-free chicken broth
- 1 teaspoon dried thyme
- 1 tablespoon lemon juice
- 2 tablespoons gluten-free all-purpose flour with xanthan gum

Directions :

1. Preheat oven to 400°F.
2. Season both sides of chicken with cumin, paprika, salt, and pepper.
3. In a large ovenproof skillet over medium-high heat, melt 3 tablespoons buttery spread. Place chicken skin-side down first and sear each side of chicken until crispy brown, about 2–3 minutes each. Remove chicken from pan.
4. Add garlic to the skillet and cook for 30 seconds until fragrant. Add milk, broth, thyme, and lemon juice. Bring liquid to a low simmer.
5. Place chicken back into the skillet and transfer to oven. Roast chicken for 25–30 minutes or until fully cooked and internal temperature of chicken is 165°F.
6. Remove chicken from the skillet. Heat up milk sauce over a medium to high heat and bring to a low simmer. Whisk in remaining buttery spread and flour until flour dissolves. Cook until gravy is thick and creamy, about 2–3 minutes. Remove from heat, pour on top of chicken thighs, and serve.

Hawaiian Chicken Kebabs

- **Ingredients :**
- ⅓ cup ketchup
- ¼ cup light brown sugar, packed
- ⅓ cup gluten-free soy sauce
- ¼ cup pineapple juice
- 1½ tablespoons rice vinegar
- 1 tablespoon jarred minced garlic
- 1 tablespoon jarred minced ginger
- ½ teaspoon sesame oil
- 4 (6-ounce) boneless, skinless chicken breasts, chopped into 1¼" cubes
- 1 large red onion, peeled and diced into 1¼" pieces
- 1 large green bell pepper, seeded and diced into 1¼" pieces
- 3 cups cubed fresh pineapple
- 2 tablespoons olive oil
- ½ teaspoon salt
- ¼ ground black pepper

Directions :

1. In a small bowl, whisk together ketchup, brown sugar, soy sauce, pineapple juice, vinegar, garlic, ginger, and sesame oil.
2. Place chicken in a gallon-sized sealable plastic bag. Save ½ cup marinade in the refrigerator, then pour remaining marinade into bag with chicken. Seal bag and refrigerate 1 hour. Soak ten wooden skewer sticks in water for 1 hour.
3. Preheat a gas grill to 400°F. In a medium bowl, add red onions, bell peppers, and pineapple and drizzle with olive oil and toss. Season with salt and pepper. Thread marinated chicken, onions, bell peppers, and pineapple onto skewers.
4. Place skewers on a greased grill. Grill 5 minutes, then brush marinade along tops with reserved ¼ cup marinade. Turn skewers over and brush remaining ¼ cup marinade on opposite side.
5. Grill 4–5 more minutes, or until chicken registers 165°F on a meat thermometer. Serve warm.

Teriyaki Chicken

Ingredients :
- 1 tablespoon vegetable oil
- 1 pound boneless, skinless chicken thighs, cut into 1½" pieces
- 1 teaspoon cornstarch
- 2 teaspoons water
- ¼ cup gluten-free soy sauce
- 3 tablespoons light brown sugar, packed
- 1 tablespoon honey
- 3 tablespoons rice wine vinegar
- 1 tablespoon jarred minced garlic
- 1 teaspoon jarred minced ginger
- 1 tablespoon sesame oil

Directions :

1. Heat vegetable oil in a large skillet over medium heat. Cook chicken for 6–8 minutes, stirring occasionally, until lightly browned and crisp.
2. In a small bowl, whisk together cornstarch and water. In another small bowl, whisk together soy sauce, brown sugar, honey, vinegar, ginger, sesame oil, and the cornstarch mixture to combine.
3. Add the garlic to the skillet, stir, and sauté for 30 seconds, until fragrant. Pour in sauce and stir to coat chicken. Simmer for 2–3 minutes until sauce thickens.

Baked Honey Mustard Chicken

Ingredients :
- 4 (6-ounce) boneless, skinless chicken breasts

- ½ teaspoon salt
- ¼ teaspoon ground black pepper
- 1 tablespoon olive oil
- ¼ cup stone-ground mustard
- 2 tablespoons Dijon mustard
- ½ cup honey
- 2 tablespoons dairy-free buttery spread

Directions :

1. Preheat oven to 375°F. Spray a 9" × 13" baking dish with gluten-free nonstick cooking spray.

2. Season chicken with salt and pepper. Heat oil in a large skillet over medium-high heat. Sear chicken on both sides until golden brown, 2–3 minutes per side.

3. In a small bowl, whisk together mustards, honey, and buttery spread. Pour half of the sauce into prepared baking pan. Top with chicken, then pour rest of sauce over top of chicken.

4. Cover with aluminum foil, then bake for 20 minutes. Uncover and bake for 10 more minutes or until chicken measures 165°F on a meat thermometer.

Pasta Primavera with Chicken

Ingredients :

- 1 (12-ounce) box gluten-free penne pasta
- 2 tablespoons plus ¼ cup olive oil, divided
- 2 (6-ounce) boneless, skinless chicken breasts
- ½ teaspoon salt
- ¼ teaspoon ground black pepper
- 1 teaspoon jarred minced garlic
- ½ medium red onion, peeled and sliced
- 1 large carrot, peeled and sliced into matchsticks
- 1 medium red bell pepper, seeded and sliced into matchsticks
- 1 medium yellow squash, sliced and halved
- 1 large zucchini, sliced and halved
- 1 cup halved grape tomatoes
- 1 tablespoon Italian seasoning
- 1 tablespoon lemon juice

Directions :

1. Cook pasta according to the package directions.

2. Heat 2 tablespoons of olive oil in a large skillet over medium-high heat. Add chicken and season with salt and black pepper. Cook for 6–7 minutes on each side until golden and cooked through and a meat thermometer reaches 165°F. Remove from the skillet and let rest 10 minutes before slicing.

3. Add the ¼ cup of olive oil and garlic to the skillet and sauté for 30 seconds until fragrant. Add red onions, carrots, and bell peppers and sauté 2 minutes. Add squash and zucchini and sauté 2 minutes until softened. Add tomatoes, Italian seasoning, and lemon juice and sauté 2 minutes longer.

4. Toss pasta with the vegetable mixture in a large bowl to combine. Top with sliced chicken and serve.

Chicken and Dumplings

Ingredients :

CHICKEN
- 4 cups gluten-free chicken broth
- 4 cups diced cooked skinless chicken breasts
- 2 cups frozen mixed vegetables
- 1 tablespoon dried sage
- 1 tablespoon dried thyme
- 1 tablespoon onion powder
- ½ teaspoon salt
- 2 cups unsweetened almond milk
- 6 tablespoons gluten-free cornstarch

DUMPLINGS
- 2 large eggs
- 1½ cups Bisquick Gluten Free Pancake & Baking Mix
- 4 tablespoons dairy-free buttery spread, melted
- ⅔ cup unsweetened almond milk

Directions :

1. In a large pot, add chicken broth, chicken, vegetables, sage, thyme, onion powder, and salt. Bring to a low boil over medium heat.

2. In a small bowl, add milk and cornstarch together and stir until cornstarch is dissolved. Pour the milk mixture into the large pot with chicken broth and stir until fully combined. Continue to boil.

3. In a medium bowl, whisk eggs. Add Bisquick and stir. Add the buttery spread and milk to the Bisquick mixture and stir until fully combined. The batter will be sticky.

4. Using a greased ice cream scoop, drop dumpling batter into the chicken broth mixture. Reduce the heat to low and cook for 10 minutes. Cover and cook for an additional 15 minutes. Remove from heat and serve.

Buffalo Turkey Burgers

- **Ingredients :**
- 1 pound ground turkey
- 1 stalk celery, finely diced
- 2 teaspoons gluten-free and dairy-free hot wing sauce
- ½ teaspoon salt
- ¼ teaspoon ground black pepper
- 2 tablespoons olive oil

Directions :

1. In a large bowl, mix ground turkey, celery, wing sauce, salt, and pepper. Form four patties.

2. Heat olive oil in a large skillet over medium heat. Place turkey burgers in the skillet and cook on one side for 4–5 minutes until browned, then flip. Cook another 4–5 minutes or until burgers are cooked all the way through and the internal temperature is 165°F.

Easy Chicken Fried Rice

- **Ingredients :**
- 3 tablespoons sesame oil
- 2 (6-ounce) boneless, skinless chicken breasts, diced into 1" pieces
- 1 tablespoon jarred minced garlic
- 2 tablespoons jarred minced ginger
- 1 cup frozen peas
- ½ cup peeled and diced carrots
- 6 large eggs, whisked
- 3 cups cooked white rice
- 3 tablespoons gluten-free soy sauce

Directions :

1. Add oil to a large skillet or wok and heat over medium-high heat. Add chicken and cook for 3–5 minutes, flipping so all sides cook evenly.

2. Add garlic, ginger, peas, and carrots and cook for 2 minutes.

3. Push the chicken mixture to one side of the skillet, then add eggs and scramble for 1–2 minutes. Stir eggs and the chicken mixture together.

4. Add rice to the skillet and stir to combine with the chicken mixture.

5. Pour soy sauce over rice and stir to combine. Fry the rice for another 3–5 minutes. Serve warm.

Chicken Marsala

- **Ingredients :**
- ½ cup gluten-free all-purpose flour with xanthan gum

- ¼ cup gluten-free cornstarch
- ½ teaspoon salt
- ¼ teaspoon ground black pepper
- 3 (6-ounce) boneless, skinless chicken breasts cut into ½" pieces
- 2 tablespoons olive oil
- 1 teaspoon jarred minced garlic
- 1 tablespoon onion powder
- 2 cups sliced white button mushrooms
- ½ cup Marsala wine
- ½ cup gluten-free chicken broth
- 2 tablespoons dairy-free buttery spread

Directions :

1. Preheat oven to 200°F. Line a baking sheet with aluminum foil and spray with gluten-free nonstick cooking spray.
2. Add flour, cornstarch, salt, and pepper to a pie pan and whisk to combine. Dredge chicken pieces in flour.
3. Heat olive oil in a large skillet over medium-high heat. Pan-fry chicken for 3 minutes on each side until golden brown. Place chicken onto prepared baking sheet and place in the oven to keep warm. Drain most of the oil from the skillet, reserving 1 tablespoon in the skillet.
4. Add garlic and onion powder to the skillet and sauté for 30 seconds until fragrant. Add mushrooms to the skillet and sauté for 5 minutes until nicely browned. Pour Marsala and broth into the skillet and simmer for 1 minute to reduce sauce slightly. Stir in the buttery spread and return chicken to the skillet and simmer for 5 more minutes until sauce is reduced and slightly thickened.

Melt-in-Your-Mouth Chicken Breasts

- **Ingredients :**
- 1 cup mayonnaise
- 1 tablespoon seasoned salt
- 4 (6-ounce) boneless, skinless chicken breasts, sliced in half

Directions :

1. Preheat oven to 375°F. Spray a 9" × 13" baking dish with gluten-free nonstick cooking spray.
2. In a small bowl, mix mayonnaise and salt together.
3. Place chicken in the dish and spread with the mayonnaise mixture.
4. Bake for 45 minutes until the internal temperature is 165°F.

Easy Homemade Chicken Nuggets

- **Ingredients :**
- ¾ cup gluten-free all-purpose flour with xanthan gum
- ½ cup gluten-free bread crumbs
- 1 tablespoon paprika
- ½ teaspoon garlic
- ½ teaspoon salt
- 4 (6-ounce) boneless, skinless chicken breasts, cut into 1½" pieces
- 1 large egg, beaten
- ¼ cup dairy-free buttery spread, melted

Directions :

1. Preheat oven to 450°F. Spray a baking sheet with gluten-free nonstick cooking spray.
2. Place flour, bread crumbs, paprika, garlic, and salt in a large sealable plastic bag. Place chicken and egg in a large bowl and stir until pieces are fully covered in egg.
3. Place chicken in the plastic bag with the flour mixture and toss to coat.
4. Place coated chicken on the greased baking sheet. Drizzle buttery spread over chicken. Bake for 20 minutes until golden brown.

Baked Bacon Ranch Chicken Breasts

- **Ingredients :**
- 1 cup mayonnaise
- 1 tablespoon dried dill
- 1½ teaspoons garlic powder
- 1½ teaspoons onion powder
- 2 teaspoons dried parsley
- 1½ teaspoons salt
- ½ teaspoon ground black pepper
- 1 tablespoon granulated sugar
- 4 (6-ounce) boneless, skinless chicken breasts, sliced in half
- ½ cup crumbled cooked gluten-free bacon

Directions :

1. Preheat oven to 375°F. Spray a 9" × 13" baking dish with gluten-free nonstick cooking spray.
2. In a small bowl, mix mayonnaise, seasonings, and sugar together.
3. Place chicken in the dish and spread with the mayonnaise mixture.
4. Bake for 45 minutes until the internal temperature is 165°F. Remove from oven and top with crumbled bacon before serving.

Chicken Fajitas

- **Ingredients :**
- 3 tablespoons olive oil, divided
- 2 tablespoons lime juice
- 2 tablespoons ground cumin
- 1 teaspoon garlic powder
- 1 teaspoon paprika
- 1 tablespoon dried oregano
- 1 teaspoon salt
- 2 (6-ounce) boneless, skinless chicken breasts, cut into thin strips
- 3 large red, green, and yellow bell peppers, seeded and cut into strips
- 1 large sweet onion, peeled and thinly sliced

Directions :

1. In a large bowl, combine 2 tablespoons olive oil, lime juice, and seasonings, then add the chicken. Toss chicken to coat; cover and marinate in the refrigerator for 30 minutes.

2. In a large skillet over medium-high heat, heat remaining 1 tablespoon oil, then sauté peppers and onions for 5 minutes until soft. Remove from skillet and keep warm.

3. In the same skillet, cook marinated chicken over medium-high heat for 5–6 minutes or until no longer pink. Return peppers and onions to skillet and cook for another 5–6 minutes before serving.

Bruschetta Chicken Bake

Ingredients :

CHICKEN
- 6 large Roma tomatoes, diced
- ½ cup chopped fresh basil
- 1 tablespoon jarred minced garlic
- 2 teaspoons light brown sugar, packed
- 2 tablespoons balsamic vinegar
- 1 teaspoon salt, divided
- 4 (6-ounce) boneless, skinless chicken breasts
- ¼ teaspoon ground black pepper

GLAZE
- 1 cup balsamic vinegar
- ½ cup granulated sugar
- 2 tablespoons honey
- ½ teaspoon salt

Directions :

1. Preheat oven to 375°F and spray a 9" × 13" baking dish with gluten-free nonstick cooking spray.

2. In a large bowl, toss tomatoes, basil, garlic, brown sugar, vinegar, and ½ teaspoon salt.

3. Lay chicken breasts flat in the bottom of the baking dish and season with remaining salt and pepper. Pour the tomato mixture over chicken.

4. Bake for 35–45 minutes or until chicken reaches an internal temperature of 165°F.

5. While chicken is baking, add the glaze ingredients to a medium saucepan. Bring to a boil over medium-high heat, then reduce to medium-low heat and allow to simmer 10–15 minutes. The sauce should reduce by half. Remove from heat.

6. Remove chicken from the oven when done and drizzle with glaze.

Homestyle Chicken and Rice Casserole

Ingredients :
- 12 tablespoons dairy-free buttery spread, divided
- 1 cup chopped white button mushrooms
- 1 cup chopped celery
- ½ teaspoon jarred minced garlic
- ½ cup gluten-free all-purpose flour with xanthan gum
- 1 teaspoon dried thyme
- 1 teaspoon onion powder
- 3 cups gluten-free chicken broth
- ½ teaspoon salt
- ⅛ teaspoon ground black pepper
- ⅛ teaspoon ground nutmeg
- 1½ cups unsweetened almond milk
- 4 (6-ounce) boneless, skinless chicken breasts, cubed
- 2 cups water
- 2 cups instant white rice

Directions :

1. Preheat oven to 400°F. Spray a 9" × 13" baking pan with gluten-free nonstick cooking spray.

2. In a large skillet, heat 4 tablespoons buttery spread over medium-high heat; sauté mushrooms, celery, and garlic until tender, about 2–3 minutes. Sprinkle with flour, thyme, and onion powder. Stir to coat vegetables. Stir in broth, salt, pepper, and nutmeg. Stir the mixture until flour dissolves. Bring soup to a boil and stir for 2 minutes until thickened. Reduce the heat to a low simmer and stir in milk. Simmer uncovered for 10–15 minutes. Add chicken, water, and rice to the mixture and stir to combine.

3. Pour the mixture into prepared baking pan. Place remaining buttery spread evenly over the top of the

chicken mixture.

4. Bake for 60 minutes to 75 minutes until rice is tender and chicken is cooked through. Cool 15 minutes before serving.

Honey Lemon Ginger Chicken

Ingredients :
- 2 teaspoons sesame oil, divided
- 1½ teaspoons jarred minced garlic
- 1 tablespoon jarred minced ginger
- ¼ teaspoon salt
- ½ cup honey
- 4 tablespoons lemon juice
- ½ teaspoon lemon zest
- 1 tablespoon apple cider vinegar
- 1 tablespoon gluten-free soy sauce
- 3 teaspoons cornstarch
- 4 (6-ounce) boneless, skinless chicken breasts, diced
- ¼ cup peeled and shredded carrots
- ¼ cup chopped cashews

Directions :

1. In a medium saucepan, add 1 teaspoon sesame oil, garlic, and ginger. Sauté over medium heat for 2–3 minutes. Add salt, honey, lemon juice, lemon zest, vinegar, soy sauce, and cornstarch. Bring to a boil and then reduce to a simmer. Simmer to thicken while cooking chicken.

2. Heat remaining sesame oil in a large skillet over medium-high heat. Sauté chicken for about 5–8 minutes until lightly browned and no longer has pink in centers. Add carrots and cashews. Add sauce to chicken and toss to coat. Simmer for 2–3 minutes.

Easy Baked Lemon Pepper Chicken

Ingredients :
- 4 (6-ounce) boneless, skinless chicken breasts
- 1 tablespoon lemon pepper seasoning
- 1 tablespoon olive oil
- 3 tablespoons dairy-free buttery spread, melted
- 1 teaspoon jarred minced garlic
- ¼ cup gluten-free chicken broth
- ¼ cup lemon juice
- 1 tablespoon chopped fresh parsley

Directions :

1. Preheat oven to 400°F and spray a 9" × 13" baking dish with gluten-free nonstick cooking spray.
2. Season chicken on both sides with lemon pepper seasoning.
3. Heat olive oil in a large skillet over medium-high heat. Add chicken and cook for 3–5 minutes on each side until browned. Transfer chicken to prepared baking dish.
4. In a small bowl, mix together buttery spread, garlic, chicken broth, and lemon juice. Pour the buttery spread mixture over chicken.
5. Bake for 25–30 minutes until internal temperature reaches 165°F. Spoon sauce from the pan over chicken and sprinkle with parsley.

Southern Chicken-Fried Steak

Ingredients :

STEAK
- 1 cup gluten-free all-purpose flour with xanthan gum
- ½ cup cornstarch
- 2 tablespoons seasoned salt
- 4 (4-ounce) cube steaks
- ¼ teaspoon salt
- ⅛ teaspoon ground black pepper
- 2 large eggs
- ½ cup unsweetened almond milk
- ¾ cup vegetable oil

GRAVY
- 6 tablespoons gluten-free all-purpose flour with xanthan gum
- 3 cups unsweetened almond milk
- ½ teaspoon seasoned salt
- ¼ teaspoon ground black pepper

Directions :

1. Combine flour, cornstarch, and seasoned salt in a pie pan. Sprinkle both sides of steaks with salt and pepper, then place in the flour mixture. Turn to coat. Whisk eggs and milk together in a separate pie pan. Place steaks into the egg mixture, turning to coat. Place steaks back in flour and turn to coat. Place breaded meat on a clean plate.
2. Heat oil in a large skillet over medium-high heat. Add two steaks to hot oil and fry until browned, about 3–5 minutes per side. Remove each steak to a paper towel–lined plate to drain and cover with aluminum foil to keep warm. Repeat with remaining steaks.
3. After all the meat is cooked, pour the grease into a heatproof bowl. Add 2 tablespoons of grease back

to the skillet and heat over a medium-low heat.

4. Whisk flour with grease until a paste forms. Pour in the milk, whisking constantly. Add seasoned salt and pepper and cook for 5–10 minutes, whisking, until gravy is smooth and thick. Serve steaks topped with gravy.

Mongolian Beef

Ingredients :
- 1 pound flank steak, sliced thin
- ¼ cup cornstarch
- 3 tablespoons vegetable oil
- ⅓ cup gluten-free soy sauce
- ½ cup light brown sugar, packed
- ¼ cup water
- 1 tablespoon jarred minced ginger
- 1 tablespoon jarred minced garlic
- 2 green onions, sliced for garnish

Directions :

1. In a large sealable plastic bag, add steak and cornstarch and keep turning over the bag until meat is fully coated.

2. Heat oil in a large skillet over high heat. Add steak in a single layer and cook on each side for 1 minute until the edges are starting to brown. Remove and set aside on a plate.

3. In a small bowl, combine soy sauce, brown sugar, water, ginger, and garlic. Add sauce to the skillet and bring to a boil. Add steak back to the skillet and allow sauce to thicken for 2–3 minutes. Toss with green onions.

Brown Butter Filet Mignon

Ingredients :
- 1 (6-ounce) filet mignon
- ½ teaspoon salt
- 1 tablespoon olive oil
- 1 tablespoon dairy-free buttery spread
- 1 teaspoon dried sage

Directions :

1. Cover fillet on both sides with salt and allow steak to come to room temperature.

2. In a small sauté pan, heat olive oil over high heat until 350°F. (The oil needs to be really hot to make a perfect crust.)

3. Place fillet in the pan and cook over high heat for 3 minutes. Turn steak over and add buttery spread and sage. Spoon buttery spread and sage from the pan over steak as it cooks for 3 more minutes. Remove steak from the pan and allow it to rest before serving.

Cottage Pie

Ingredients :
- ½ cup dairy-free buttery spread, divided
- 1 medium sweet onion, peeled and chopped
- 1½ pounds 90/10 ground round beef
- 1 teaspoon gluten-free Worcestershire sauce
- 2 teaspoons salt, divided
- ¼ teaspoon ground black pepper
- 1 teaspoon dried thyme
- ½ teaspoon dried rosemary
- ½ cup gluten-free beef broth
- 2 cups mixed frozen vegetables, such as corn, peas, and carrots
- 3 large potatoes, peeled, quartered, and boiled

Directions :
1. Preheat oven to 400°F. Spray a 9" × 13" baking dish with gluten-free nonstick cooking spray.
2. In a large skillet, melt 4 tablespoons buttery spread over medium heat. Add onions and cook for 5–10 minutes until tender.
3. Add ground beef and Worcestershire sauce. Season with 1 teaspoon salt, pepper, thyme, and rosemary. Cook for 3–5 minutes until beef is no longer pink. Add beef broth and mixed vegetables and simmer for 10 minutes.
4. Add boiled potatoes and remaining buttery spread and salt in a large bowl and mash with a potato masher or hand mixer.
5. Spread the beef mixture in an even layer in prepared baking dish. Spread mashed potatoes over the top of the beef mixture. Use a fork to poke the surface all over the top of the potatoes.
6. Bake for 30 minutes until browned and bubbling. Broil for 1–2 minutes to brown the mashed potatoes before serving.

Mini Meatloaves

Ingredients :
- 1 pound 90/10 ground beef
- 1 tablespoon onion powder
- 1 teaspoon garlic powder

- 1 teaspoon salt
- 2 tablespoons gluten-free Worcestershire sauce
- ½ cup gluten-free bread crumbs
- 1 large egg, whisked
- ¼ cup unsweetened almond milk
- ¼ cup light brown sugar, packed
- 1 teaspoon mustard
- ⅓ cup ketchup

Directions :

1. Preheat oven to 350°F and spray a twelve-cup muffin tin with gluten-free nonstick cooking spray.
2. In a large bowl, combine beef, seasonings, Worcestershire sauce, bread crumbs, egg, and milk. Press mixture into muffin tin.
3. In a small bowl, whisk brown sugar, mustard, and ketchup. Spoon sauce over the meat.
4. Bake for 30 minutes until internal temperature reaches 160°F. Remove from muffin tin and serve.

Sautéed Beef with Broccoli

Ingredients :

- ½ cup gluten-free soy sauce
- ¼ cup cornstarch
- 3 tablespoons rice wine vinegar
- 3 tablespoons light brown sugar, packed
- 1 tablespoon gluten-free peanut butter
- 1 tablespoon jarred minced ginger
- 1 tablespoon jarred minced garlic
- 1 pound flank steak, sliced thin
- 2 teaspoons sesame oil
- 2 cups broccoli florets
- ¼ cup gluten-free beef broth

Directions :

1. In a small bowl, mix together soy sauce, cornstarch, vinegar, brown sugar, peanut butter, ginger, and garlic. Pour half the liquid over sliced meat in a bowl and toss. Reserve the other half of the sauce and set aside.
2. Heat oil in a large skillet or wok over high heat. Add broccoli and stir-fry for 1 minute. Remove to a plate.
3. Add meat in a single layer and cook for 1 minute. Turn meat over and cook for another 30 seconds. Remove to a plate.
4. Pour reserved sauce and beef broth into the skillet. Stir and cook for 2–3 minutes until sauce starts to

thicken. Add beef and broccoli back to the skillet and toss to coat and simmer for another 2 minutes.

Swedish Meatballs

Ingredients :

MEATBALLS
- 1 pound 90/10 ground beef
- ⅓ cup gluten-free bread crumbs
- ¼ teaspoon ground allspice
- ¼ teaspoon ground nutmeg
- 1 teaspoon onion powder
- 1 teaspoon garlic powder
- ½ teaspoon salt
- ⅛ teaspoon ground black pepper
- 1 large egg, whisked
- ½ cup unsweetened almond milk
- 2 tablespoons olive oil

SAUCE
- 2 tablespoons dairy-free buttery spread
- 4 tablespoons gluten-free all-purpose flour with xanthan gum
- 2 cups gluten-free beef broth
- 1 cup unsweetened almond milk
- ½ teaspoon salt
- ¼ teaspoon ground black pepper
- 1 tablespoon gluten-free Worcestershire sauce
- 1 teaspoon Dijon mustard

Directions :

1. In a medium bowl, combine beef, bread crumbs, allspice, nutmeg, onion powder, garlic powder, salt, pepper, egg, and milk. Mix until combined.

2. Roll meat into twenty-four small meatballs. In a large skillet, heat olive oil over medium-high heat. Add meatballs and cook for 7–12 minutes, turning to brown on each side and to cook throughout. Transfer to a plate and cover with aluminum foil.

3. Add buttery spread to the skillet and melt. Whisk in flour until it dissolves and turns brown. Pour in broth, milk, salt, pepper, Worcestershire sauce, and mustard. Stir to combine ingredients. Bring to a simmer. Add meatballs back to the skillet and simmer for another 1–2 minutes.

Easy Homemade Beef Stroganoff

Ingredients :
- 1½ pounds beef round steak, cut into thin strips
- ½ teaspoon salt, divided
- 4 tablespoons dairy-free buttery spread
- 1 medium sweet onion, peeled and sliced
- 1 teaspoon jarred minced garlic
- 2 cups sliced white button mushrooms
- 4 tablespoons gluten-free all-purpose flour with xanthan gum
- 1 cup unsweetened almond milk
- ¼ teaspoon ground black pepper
- 1 tablespoon gluten-free Worcestershire sauce
- 1 teaspoon Dijon mustard
- 2 cups gluten-free beef broth
- ½ cup dairy-free sour cream

Directions :

1. Sprinkle steak strips with ¼ teaspoon salt. Heat buttery spread in a large skillet over medium-high heat and add steak and quickly brown for 1 minute. Remove steak and place on a plate. Add onions, garlic, and mushrooms to the skillet. Sauté for 2 minutes until tender.

2. Sprinkle the skillet with flour. Put steak back into the skillet with onion and mushrooms. Add milk, remaining salt, pepper, Worcestershire sauce, Dijon mustard, and beef broth and stir to combine. Cook covered for 15 minutes.

3. Stir in sour cream the last few minutes, right before you serve.

Stuffed Peppers

Ingredients :
- 2 tablespoons olive oil
- 1 small sweet onion, peeled and diced
- 1 tablespoon jarred minced garlic
- ½ pound 90/10 ground beef
- ½ pound gluten-free Italian sausage
- 2 (8-ounce) cans tomato sauce, divided
- ½ cup white rice, uncooked
- 1¼ cups water
- 1 tablespoon gluten-free Worcestershire sauce
- 1 cup gluten-free beef broth
- 6 green bell peppers, cut in half, with stem and seeds removed
- 1 tablespoon Italian seasoning

Directions :

1. Preheat oven to 350°F. Spray a 9" × 13" baking dish with gluten-free nonstick cooking spray.

2. Heat olive oil in large skillet on medium-high heat and add the onions and garlic and cook for 1–2 minutes. Add in beef and sausage and cook for 3–5 minutes until brown and crumbled.

3. Stir in one can of tomato sauce, rice, water, and Worcestershire sauce. Bring to a simmer, reduce heat, and cover. Cook 15–20 minutes or until rice is tender.

4. Pour broth into the baking dish. Fill each pepper with the rice mixture and place in prepared dish. Mix remaining can of tomato sauce and Italian seasoning in a bowl and pour over stuffed peppers. Cover with aluminum foil and bake 1 hour.

Salisbury Steak

Ingredients :

PATTIES
- 1 pound 90/10 ground beef
- ¼ cup gluten-free bread crumbs
- 1 large egg, beaten
- 1 tablespoon gluten-free Worcestershire sauce
- 1 teaspoon onion powder
- ½ teaspoon garlic powder
- ¼ teaspoon salt
- ¼ teaspoon ground black pepper
- 2 tablespoons olive oil
- 2 tablespoons dairy-free buttery spread
- 1 tablespoon jarred minced garlic
- 1½ cups sliced white button mushrooms
- 1 small sweet onion, peeled and thinly sliced

GRAVY
- 1 tablespoon cornstarch
- 2 tablespoons cold water
- 2 cups gluten-free beef broth
- 2 tablespoons ketchup
- 2 tablespoons gluten-free Worcestershire sauce

Directions :

1. In a large bowl, mix together beef, bread crumbs, egg, Worcestershire sauce, onion powder, garlic powder, salt, and pepper. Shape into four oval patties.

2. Heat olive oil in a large skillet over medium-high heat. Cook patties for 5–6 minutes on each side and then remove from the skillet.

3. Add buttery spread, garlic, mushrooms, and onions to the skillet and cook for 5–10 minutes until onions are golden and mushrooms are softened.

4. In a small bowl, mix cornstarch with cold water. Add beef broth, ketchup, Worcestershire sauce, and the cornstarch mixture to the skillet and whisk until smooth.

5. Reduce heat to medium, stirring often, and simmer for 1–2 minutes until gravy starts to thicken. Add patties back into the skillet and cook for 5 minutes.

Oven-Baked St. Louis–Style Ribs

Ingredients :
- 1 tablespoon gluten-free liquid smoke
- 1 tablespoon Dijon mustard
- ½ teaspoon apple cider vinegar
- 4 pounds St. Louis–style ribs, membranes removed
- 1 tablespoon garlic powder
- 1 tablespoon onion powder
- 2 tablespoons light brown sugar, packed
- 1 teaspoon paprika
- 1 teaspoon seasoning salt
- ½ tablespoon dry mustard
- 2 cups gluten-free barbecue sauce

Directions :

1. Preheat oven to 325°F. Line a baking sheet with aluminum foil and spray with gluten-free nonstick cooking spray.

2. In a small bowl, mix liquid smoke, mustard, and vinegar. Rub sauce over both sides of ribs.

3. In another small bowl, mix all dry spices and seasonings and stir to combine. Sprinkle dry mix over both sides of ribs and rub into meat.

4. Place ribs on prepared baking sheet and cover with another piece of aluminum foil and seal tightly to making a pouch for ribs to cook in.

5. Bake on the middle rack for 1 hour.

6. Turn the heat down to 250°F and unwrap the ribs. Baste each side with barbecue sauce every 10 minutes for a total of 30 minutes until the internal temperature is 145°F. Allow to rest 5–10 minutes before cutting.

Beef Tenderloin

- **Ingredients :**
- 5 pounds beef tenderloin, trimmed and cut in half
- 2 teaspoons salt
- 2 teaspoons ground black pepper
- 2 tablespoons vegetable oil
- 3 tablespoons dairy-free buttery spread
- 2 teaspoons jarred minced garlic
- 1 tablespoon dried rosemary

Directions :

1. Preheat oven to 450°F. Spray a large roasting pan with gluten-free nonstick cooking spray.

2. Season each beef tenderloin roast with salt and pepper. Heat oil in a large skillet over medium-high heat until hot. Sear roasts for 3 minutes on all four sides until well browned.

3. In a small bowl, combine buttery spread, garlic, and rosemary together. Rub the buttery spread mixture on beef.

4. Transfer beef to prepared roasting pan. Roast for 20–25 minutes for medium-rare or until a meat thermometer inserted in the thickest part registers 135°F. For medium doneness, cook until thermometer reaches 145°F. (Temperature will continue to rise about 5 degrees while meat rests.) Transfer the roasts to a carving board and let rest for 15 minutes. Carve beef tenderloin into ½"-thick slices and serve.

Prime Rib

Ingredients :

- 5 pounds beef prime rib
- 2 teaspoons salt
- ½ teaspoon ground black pepper
- 4 tablespoons jarred minced garlic
- 2 teaspoons dried rosemary
- 2 teaspoons dried thyme
- ¼ cup olive oil

Directions :

1. Allow prime rib to come to room temperature for 1 hour before cooking. Season it on all sides with salt and cover it loosely with plastic wrap.

2. Preheat oven to 500°F with the rack in the lower third of the oven. In a small bowl, stir together pepper, garlic, rosemary, thyme, and olive oil. Rub all over top and sides with the herb mixture.

3. Place meat into a large roasting pan bone-side down. Bake at 500°F for 15 minutes, then reduce the oven temperature to 325°F and continue baking until desired doneness. (Note: The meat will continue to cook once it's taken out of the oven, so remove the meat from the oven 5 degrees before

it reaches your optimal temperature.)

4. For rare, cook until thermometer reaches 125°F (10–12 minutes/pound)
5. For medium-rare, cook until thermometer reaches 135°F (13–14 minutes/pound)
6. For medium, cook until thermometer reaches 145°F (14–15 minutes/pound)
7. For medium-well, cook until thermometer reaches 150°F (17–20 minutes/pound)
8. Remove meat from the oven and allow it to rest for 30 minutes before carving. Carve your roast by slicing against the grain at about ½" thickness.

Easy Bacon Burger Pie

Ingredients :
- 1 tablespoon olive oil
- 1 pound 90/10 ground beef
- 2 teaspoons seasoned salt
- 1 cup chopped cooked gluten-free bacon
- ½ cup chopped dill pickles
- ½ cup halved grape tomatoes
- ½ cup Bisquick Gluten Free Pancake & Baking Mix
- 1 cup unsweetened almond milk
- 3 large eggs, whisked

Directions :

1. Heat oven to 400°F. Spray a 9" pie pan with gluten-free nonstick cooking spray.

2. Heat oil in a large skillet and cook beef over medium-high heat for 5–7 minutes, stirring frequently, until beef is brown and crumbled; drain. Stir in seasoned salt, bacon, pickles, and tomatoes and cook for 2 minutes. Spread beef mixture in prepared pie pan.

3. In a medium bowl, stir Bisquick, milk, and eggs until combined. Pour on top of the beef mixture.

4. Bake 25–30 minutes until a knife inserted in the center comes out clean.

Taco Beef

Ingredients :
- 1 teaspoon olive oil
- 1 pound 90/10 ground beef
- 1 tablespoon ground cumin
- 2 teaspoons onion powder
- ½ teaspoon garlic powder
- 2 teaspoons paprika
- 2 teaspoons dried oregano
- ½ teaspoon salt

Directions :

1. Heat olive oil in a large skillet over medium heat and cook beef 6–8 minutes until browned and crumbled; drain excess oil.

2. In a small bowl, mix seasonings together.

3. Stir seasoning mix into beef and simmer for 2 minutes until heated through.

Korean Beef

Ingredients :
- 1 tablespoon vegetable oil
- 1 pound 90/10 ground beef
- 2 teaspoons jarred minced garlic
- ¼ cup light brown sugar, packed
- ¼ cup gluten-free soy sauce
- 2 teaspoons sesame oil
- ½ teaspoon jarred minced ginger
- ¼ teaspoon crushed red pepper flakes
- 2 green onions, thinly sliced
- ¼ teaspoon sesame seeds
- 4 cups cooked rice

Directions :

1. Heat vegetable oil in a large skillet over medium heat and cook beef and garlic for 6–8 minutes until beef is browned and crumbled.

2. In a small bowl, mix brown sugar, soy sauce, sesame oil, ginger, and red pepper flakes.

3. Stir sauce into beef and simmer for 2 minutes until heated through. Sprinkle with green onions and sesame seeds. Serve over rice.

Pork Chop Suey

Ingredients :
- 3 tablespoons vegetable oil
- 1 pound pork tenderloin, cut into 1½" strips
- 1 cup peeled and diced sweet onion
- 1 cup sliced white button mushrooms
- 1 cup diced celery
- 1 teaspoon jarred minced ginger
- 1 cup gluten-free chicken broth
- ½ teaspoon salt

- ½ teaspoon ground black pepper
- 1 (14.5-ounce) can bean sprouts, drained and rinsed
- 1 (5-ounce) can water chestnuts, drained and sliced
- 5 (5-ounce) cans bamboo shoots
- 2 teaspoons cornstarch
- ⅓ cup water
- ¼ cup gluten-free soy sauce
- 1 teaspoon granulated sugar

Directions :

1. Heat oil in a large skillet over medium-high heat and sear pork 2–3 minutes, then add onions and mushroom and sauté for 5 minutes. Add celery, ginger, chicken broth, salt, and pepper, cover and simmer for 5 minutes. Add sprouts, water chestnuts, and bamboo shoots. Bring to a boil.

2. In a small bowl, combine cornstarch, water, soy sauce, and sugar. Mix together and add to skillet. Cook for 5 minutes until thickened.

Italian Meatballs

Ingredients :
- 1 cup gluten-free bread crumbs
- 2 tablespoons jarred minced garlic
- 2 tablespoons Italian seasoning
- 1 tablespoon onion powder
- 1 teaspoon salt
- ¾ cup unsweetened almond milk
- 2 pounds 90/10 ground beef
- 2 large eggs, whisked

Directions :

1. Preheat oven to 375°F. Line two baking sheets with aluminum foil and spray with gluten-free nonstick cooking spray.

2. In a small bowl, add bread crumbs, garlic, Italian seasoning, onion powder, salt, and milk and stir to fully combine.

3. In a large bowl, mix beef and eggs together. Stir in the bread crumb mixture. Form the meatball mixture into thirty-six 2" balls and place onto prepared baking sheets.

4. Bake for 20–25 minutes until browned and cooked through.

Southwestern Tamale Pie

- **Ingredients :**
- 1 teaspoon olive oil
- 1½ pounds 90/10 ground beef
- 1 small sweet onion, peeled and chopped
- ½ cup seeded and chopped green bell pepper
- 1 teaspoon jarred minced garlic
- 1 (14.5-ounce) can diced tomatoes, including liquid
- 1 (8-ounce) can tomato sauce
- 1 (11-ounce) can corn, drained
- ½ cup sliced black olives
- 1 teaspoon salt
- 1 tablespoon chili powder
- 1 teaspoon ground cumin
- ¼ teaspoon ground black pepper
- 1½ cups unsweetened almond milk
- 1 tablespoon granulated sugar
- ½ teaspoon salt
- 2 tablespoons dairy-free buttery spread
- 1 cup gluten-free cornmeal
- 2 large eggs, whisked

Directions :

1. Preheat oven to 375°F. Spray a 9" × 13" baking pan with gluten-free nonstick cooking spray.

2. Heat olive oil in a large skillet over medium-high heat and cook beef with onions and peppers for 6–8 minutes until beef is browned and crumbled; drain oil.

3. Stir in garlic, tomatoes with juice, tomato sauce, corn, olives, salt, chili powder, cumin, and black pepper and bring to a low boil. Reduce heat to medium-low and simmer for 5 minutes. Transfer to the prepared pan.

4. In a large saucepan over medium heat, add milk, sugar, salt, and buttery spread. Reduce heat to low and stir in cornmeal, stirring constantly, until thickened.

5. Slowly add in whisked eggs, stirring until combined. Pour the milk mixture over the meat mixture, smoothing over the surface.

6. Bake 30–40 minutes until golden brown. Allow to cool for 5–10 minutes before serving.

Baked Ham with Brown Sugar Glaze

- **Ingredients :**
- 1 (10-pound) fully cooked bone-in, spiral-cut ham
- 1 (20-ounce) can pineapple tidbits with juice
- ¾ cup light brown sugar, packed

- ½ teaspoon ground cinnamon
- ¼ teaspoon ground ginger
- ¼ teaspoon ground cloves

Directions :

1. Allow ham to come to room temperature for 1–2 hours before baking.
2. In a medium saucepan over medium heat, combine pineapple, brown sugar, cinnamon, ginger, and cloves and cook for 3–5 minutes, stirring frequently.
3. Preheat oven to 300°F. Line a large roasting pan with aluminum foil and spray with gluten-free nonstick cooking spray.
4. Place ham cut-side down in prepared pan.
5. Brush 2 tablespoons glaze onto ham. Reserve remaining glaze for later. Cover ham tightly with a tent of aluminum foil. Bake at 300°F for 1½–2 hours. Remove ham from the oven and remove aluminum foil.
6. Increase the oven temperature to 400°F. Brush remaining glaze over ham. Return to the oven and continue to bake for 15 minutes until internal temperature reaches 140°F. Allow to rest for 15 minutes before slicing and serving.

Pork Tenderloin

Ingredients :
- 1 tablespoon olive oil
- 1 pound pork tenderloin
- 2 teaspoons seasoned salt
- ½ cup mayonnaise

Directions :

1. Preheat oven to 450°F. Spray a large roasting pan with gluten-free nonstick cooking spray.
2. Heat olive oil in a large skillet over medium-high heat and cook tenderloin for 10 minutes, searing each side.
3. Transfer meat to prepared roasting pan. Sprinkle seasoned salt all over tenderloin and coat with mayonnaise. Bake 20 minutes until a thermometer reads an internal temperature of 145°F.

Smothered Pork Chops

Ingredients :
- 1 cup gluten-free all-purpose flour with xanthan gum
- 2 tablespoons garlic powder

- 2 tablespoons onion powder
- ½ teaspoon cayenne pepper
- 1 teaspoon salt
- ½ teaspoon ground black pepper
- 4 (4-ounce) bone-in pork chops, ¾" thick
- ¼ cup olive oil
- ¼ teaspoon white vinegar
- ½ cup unsweetened almond milk
- 1 cup gluten-free chicken broth

Directions :

1. Add flour, garlic powder, onion powder, cayenne pepper, salt, and black pepper in a pie pan and whisk to combine. Pat pork chops dry with paper towels and then dredge them in seasoned flour, shaking off the excess.

2. In a large skillet, heat olive oil over medium heat. Place pork chops in the pan in a single layer and fry for 3 minutes on each side until golden brown. Remove pork chops from the skillet and add a teaspoon of the seasoned flour mixture to the skillet.

3. To make buttermilk, add white vinegar to milk in a small bowl and let sit for 5 minutes in the refrigerator. Whisk flour into skillet grease and then pour in chicken broth. Cook for 5 minutes to reduce and thicken slightly. Stir in buttermilk and return pork chops to the skillet, covering them with sauce. Simmer for 5 minutes before serving.

German Pork Chops

Ingredients :

- 1 teaspoon olive oil
- 4 (4-ounce) boneless pork chops
- 2 cups sauerkraut, drained
- 2 medium apples, sliced
- 1 cup peeled and chopped sweet onion
- 1 cup light brown sugar, packed
- ½ teaspoon salt
- ¼ teaspoon ground black pepper

Directions :

1. Preheat oven to 350°F. Spray a 9" × 13" baking dish with gluten-free nonstick cooking spray.

2. Heat olive oil in a large skillet over medium-high heat. Brown pork chops for 5 minutes per side. Place chops into prepared baking dish.

3. In a large bowl, mix sauerkraut, apples, onions, brown sugar, salt, and pepper. Spread sauerkraut mixture over pork chops. Cover with aluminum foil. Bake for 45 minutes until internal temperature reaches 145°F.

Honey Garlic Pork Chops

Ingredients :
- 4 (4-ounce) boneless pork chops
- ¼ teaspoon salt
- ⅛ teaspoon ground black pepper
- 1 teaspoon garlic powder
- 2 tablespoons olive oil
- 1 tablespoon dairy-free buttery spread
- 3 tablespoons jarred minced garlic
- 2 teaspoons jarred minced ginger
- ¼ cup honey
- ¼ cup water
- 2 tablespoons rice vinegar

Directions :
1. Season chops with salt, pepper, and garlic powder on both sides.
2. Heat olive oil in a large ovenproof skillet over medium-high heat. Sear chops for 4–5 minutes per side until cooked through. Transfer to a plate.
3. Reduce heat to medium. Add buttery spread, garlic, and ginger to the skillet and sauté for 30 seconds until fragrant. Stir in honey, water, and vinegar. Increase heat to medium-high and continue to cook for 3–5 minutes, stirring occasionally, until sauce reduces and thickens.
4. Add pork back into the pan and baste with the sauce. Place the skillet in the oven to broil for 2 minutes or until edges are slightly charred.

Sweet and Sour Pork

Ingredients :
- ½ cup gluten-free all-purpose flour with xanthan gum
- ½ cup gluten-free cornstarch
- 1 pound boneless pork loin, cut into 1" cubes
- 1 large egg, beaten
- 2 cups plus 1 tablespoon vegetable oil, divided
- ½ cup honey
- 6 tablespoons rice vinegar
- 4 teaspoons gluten-free soy sauce
- 3 tablespoons tomato paste
- 1 tablespoon jarred minced garlic
- 1 tablespoon jarred minced ginger
- 1 cup peeled and chopped (1" pieces) white onion
- 1 cup seeded and chopped (1" pieces) red bell pepper

- 1 cup seeded and chopped (1" pieces) green bell pepper
- 1 cup canned pineapple chunks, drained (in juice)
- 1 tablespoon cornstarch
- 2 tablespoons water
- 2 tablespoons sliced green onion
- ½ teaspoon sesame seeds

Directions :

1. Combine flour and cornstarch in a large sealable plastic bag. Add pork to a medium bowl with egg and stir to fully coat pieces. Place pork in the bag of flour mixture. Keep turning over the bag until pork is fully coated.

2. Heat 2 cups oil in a large skillet or wok over medium-high heat. Add pork to the skillet and fry for 6–8 minutes until light golden brown. Drain pork on a paper towel–lined plate. Carefully discard oil from skillet. Allow oil to completely cool before disposing.

3. In a medium bowl, combine honey, vinegar, soy sauce, and tomato paste.

4. Heat the skillet over medium-high heat and add in remaining 1 tablespoon oil. Add garlic, ginger, and onions and stir-fry for 30 seconds. Add in bell peppers and stir-fry for 1 minute. Add in pineapple and stir-fry for 1 minute. Add in pork and sauce, stir to combine, and allow sauce to come to a boil.

5. In a small bowl, whisk together cornstarch and water to make a slurry. Add slurry to the skillet, stirring constantly for 1 minute until sauce thickens. Mix the ingredients with the sauce to coat the pork. Top with green onions and sesame seeds.

Crispy Salmon Cakes

Ingredients :

DILL SAUCE
- ½ cup mayonnaise
- 1 tablespoon dried dill
- 1 teaspoon horseradish sauce
- 1 teaspoon lemon juice
- ¼ teaspoon garlic salt

SALMON CAKES
- 2 large eggs, whisked
- 1 tablespoon Old Bay Seasoning
- 1 tablespoon dried dill
- 1 cup gluten-free bread crumbs
- 2 tablespoons sweet relish

- 2 (5-ounce) cans salmon, drained
- 1 cup vegetable oil

Directions :

1. In a small bowl stir together all the ingredients for the creamy dill sauce.
2. In a medium bowl, add eggs, Old Bay Seasoning, dill, bread crumbs, and relish. Mix until all ingredients are combined.
3. Add salmon to the bread-crumb mixture and stir to combine ingredients well.
4. Form eight 1"-thick salmon cakes.
5. Heat vegetable oil in a large skillet over medium-high heat.
6. Fry cakes for 3–4 minutes on each side until golden brown. Drain on a paper towel–lined plate before serving with dipping sauce.

Cajun Catfish

Ingredients :

- ½ teaspoon ground black pepper
- ½ teaspoon ground white pepper
- 1 tablespoon garlic powder
- 1 tablespoon onion powder
- 1 tablespoon paprika
- 1 teaspoon dried parsley
- ½ teaspoon cayenne pepper
- 1 teaspoon salt
- 1 tablespoon dried oregano
- 1 tablespoon dried thyme
- ½ cup gluten-free cornmeal
- 4 (6-ounce) boneless catfish fillets
- ½ cup dairy-free buttery spread

Directions :

1. In a pie pan, mix together black pepper, white pepper, garlic powder, onion powder, paprika, parsley, cayenne pepper, salt, oregano, thyme, and cornmeal until thoroughly combined. Press catfish fillets into the spice mixture on both sides to thoroughly coat.
2. Melt buttery spread in a large cast-iron pan or skillet over high heat. Allow the pan to heat up for 2–3 minutes.
3. Add fillets to the pan. The pan will sizzle up and smoke. Cook the fillets for 2–3 minutes. Using a spatula, carefully flip fillets over and cook on the other side for another 2–3 minutes.

Fish Tacos

Ingredients :

FISH
- 1 tablespoon ground cumin
- ½ teaspoon chili powder
- ½ teaspoon garlic powder
- 1 teaspoon dried oregano
- ½ teaspoon onion powder
- 1 teaspoon paprika
- ½ teaspoon salt
- ½ teaspoon ground black pepper
- 1 pound tilapia
- 1 tablespoon olive oil

SAUCE
- ⅓ cup mayonnaise
- ¼ cup lime juice
- ½ teaspoon garlic powder
- ½ teaspoon ground cumin
- ¼ teaspoon salt
- ¼ teaspoon gluten-free and dairy-free hot sauce

TACOS
- 8 white corn tortillas

Directions :

1. Preheat oven to 400°F. Line a baking sheet with parchment paper.
2. In a small bowl, add cumin, chili powder, garlic powder, oregano, onion powder, paprika, salt, and pepper and stir to combine. Rub seasoning mix onto fish fillets. Place fish on prepared baking sheet and drizzle with olive oil. Bake for 12–15 minutes until flaky and cooked through.
3. In small bowl, whisk together mayonnaise, lime juice, garlic powder, cumin, salt, and hot sauce.
4. Heat tortillas according to package directions. Break fish into large chunks and divide among tortillas. Drizzle with sauce.

Classic Shrimp Scampi

Ingredients :
- 2 tablespoons jarred minced garlic, divided
- 1 teaspoon salt

- 3 tablespoons olive oil, divided
- 1 pound large raw shrimp, peeled and deveined
- ¼ cup white wine
- 1 tablespoon lemon juice
- ¼ cup dairy-free buttery spread
- 1 tablespoon chopped fresh parsley

Directions :

1. In a medium bowl, whisk together 1 tablespoon garlic, salt, and 1 tablespoon olive oil. Add shrimp, toss to coat, and chill for 30 minutes up to 1 hour.

2. Heat remaining olive oil in a large skillet over medium heat and cook shrimp mixture for 1 minute on each side until shrimp is pink but not fully cooked. Transfer shrimp to a plate with a slotted spoon to leave as much oil in pan as possible.

3. Add remaining garlic to the skillet and cook for 1 minute until fragrant. Add wine and lemon juice and cook for 2 minutes, stirring occasionally, until sauce is reduced by half. Add buttery spread and cook for 5 minutes. Continue stirring until buttery spread is melted and sauce is thickened.

4. Add shrimp back into the skillet. Toss shrimp to coat with sauce and cook for 2 minutes until shrimp are fully cooked and the flesh is totally pink and opaque. Garnish with parsley.

Maryland-Style Crab Cakes

Ingredients :
- 1 pound jumbo lump crabmeat
- 1 large egg, beaten
- ½ cup mayonnaise
- ½ teaspoon Dijon mustard
- 1 teaspoon gluten-free Worcestershire sauce
- 1 teaspoon Old Bay Seasoning
- ⅛ teaspoon garlic powder
- ¼ teaspoon dried parsley
- ⅛ teaspoon tarragon
- ½ cup gluten-free bread crumbs
- 6 teaspoons dairy-free buttery spread

Directions :

1. Drain crabmeat and pick through it for shells, if necessary. Try not to break up the lumps. Put crabmeat in a medium bowl and set aside.

2. In a small bowl, add egg, mayonnaise, mustard, Worcestershire sauce, Old Bay Seasoning, garlic powder, parsley, and tarragon and stir to combine ingredients. Add bread crumbs to the mixture and stir to combine.

3. Gently stir the wet mixture into crabmeat, one spoonful at a time; avoid breaking up lump meat. Do not overmix.

4. Gently form the mixture into six crab cakes. Lightly grease the bottom of a baking sheet with gluten-free nonstick cooking spray and place crab cakes on prepared sheet. Place 1 teaspoon buttery spread on top of each of the cakes.

5. Broil crab cakes on low for 12–15 minutes until golden brown and cooked through. If they are browning too fast, lower the oven rack so that crab cakes can still cook for the allotted time. Remove crab cakes from the oven and allow to cool slightly before serving them.

Country Shrimp and Grits

- **Ingredients :**
- 4 cups cooked gluten-free, dairy-free grits
- 1 pound raw shrimp, peeled and deveined
- 1 tablespoon olive oil
- ½ cup chopped gluten-free bacon
- ¼ cup peeled and chopped sweet onion
- 2 tablespoons seeded and chopped green bell pepper
- 1 teaspoon jarred minced garlic
- 2 tablespoons white wine
- 1 cup unsweetened almond milk
- ½ teaspoon salt
- ¼ teaspoon ground black pepper
- 2 tablespoons gluten-free all-purpose flour with xanthan gum

Directions :

1. Cook grits according to the package directions; set aside and keep warm.

2. Rinse shrimp and pat dry. In a large skillet, heat olive oil over medium heat and fry bacon for 2–3 minutes on each side until browned; remove to a paper towel–lined plate. Drain the skillet, reserving 1 tablespoon of bacon grease in the skillet. Add onions, bell peppers, and garlic and sauté 2–3 minutes until onions are translucent.

3. Add shrimp and sauté for 4–5 minutes or until pink. Remove the shrimp mixture from the skillet, set aside, and cover to keep warm. Add white wine to the skillet and cook for 30 seconds to deglaze.

4. Add milk, salt, black pepper, and flour to a small bowl or glass measuring cup and whisk together until flour dissolves. Slowly pour the milk mixture into the skillet, stirring, and let reduce for 2–3 minutes until thickened. Serve the shrimp mixture and gravy over cooked grits.

Honey Soy–Glazed Salmon

Ingredients :
- 1 cup gluten-free soy sauce
- ¼ cup honey
- 2 tablespoons lemon juice
- 1 tablespoon jarred minced ginger
- 1 tablespoon jarred minced garlic
- 4 (4-ounce) salmon fillets

Directions :

1. In a large bowl, whisk soy sauce, honey, lemon juice, ginger, and garlic together until honey dissolves. Place salmon fillets in marinade skin-side up. Cover the bowl with plastic wrap and marinate for 30 minutes in the refrigerator.

2. Preheat broiler to high. Put salmon on an aluminum foil–lined baking sheet sprayed with gluten-free nonstick cooking spray. Place under the broiler skin-side down and broil without turning for 7–10 minutes until fish is well caramelized and is cooked through.

Steamed Mussels with Marsala Wine and Garlic

Ingredients :
- 2 tablespoons olive oil
- 1 tablespoon jarred minced garlic
- 1 small onion, peeled and thinly sliced
- 4 pounds mussels, rinsed
- ½ cup Marsala cooking wine
- ¼ cup lemon juice
- 1 cup gluten-free chicken broth

Directions :

1. Heat oil in a 6- to 8-quart stockpot over medium-high heat. Sauté garlic and onions for 1–2 minutes. Add mussels and toss.

2. Add wine, lemon juice, and chicken broth; cover the pot and steam over medium-high heat for 5–7 minutes until mussels open. Serve with broth.

Cajun Jambalaya

Ingredients :
- 3 tablespoons olive oil, divided
- 2 (6-ounce) boneless, skinless chicken breasts, cut into 1" pieces
- 1 pound gluten-free andouille sausage, thinly sliced
- 1 small green bell pepper, seeded and diced

- 1 small red bell pepper, seeded and diced
- 1 cup diced celery
- 1 small white onion, peeled and diced
- 2 tablespoons jarred minced garlic
- 1 (14-ounce) can crushed tomatoes, including liquid
- 3 cups gluten-free chicken broth
- 1½ cups uncooked white rice
- 2 tablespoons Cajun seasoning
- 1 teaspoon dried thyme
- ¼ teaspoon cayenne pepper
- 1 bay leaf
- 1 pound raw large shrimp, peeled and deveined
- 1 cup thinly sliced okra
- 2 teaspoons salt
- ¼ teaspoon ground black pepper

Directions :

1. Heat 1 tablespoon oil in a large stockpot over medium-high heat. Add chicken and sausage and sauté for 5–7 minutes, stirring occasionally, until chicken is cooked through and sausage is lightly browned. Transfer to a plate.

2. Add remaining 2 tablespoons oil to the stockpot and add bell peppers, celery, onions, and garlic. Sauté the mixture for 6 minutes, stirring occasionally, until onions are softened.

3. Add tomatoes, chicken broth, rice, Cajun seasoning, thyme, cayenne pepper, and bay leaf and stir to combine. Bring the mixture to a simmer. Reduce heat to medium-low, cover, and simmer for about 25–30 minutes until rice is nearly cooked through, stirring every 5 minutes to keep rice from burning. Add shrimp and okra and stir to combine. Continue to simmer for 5–6 minutes until shrimp are cooked through and pink. Stir in chicken, sausage, salt, and pepper. Remove and discard bay leaf. Remove from heat and serve warm.

Stuffed Jumbo Shrimp

Ingredients :
- 1 tablespoon olive oil
- ¼ cup minced celery
- 1 tablespoon jarred minced garlic
- ½ cup peeled and minced onion
- 20 fresh jumbo shrimp, peeled and deveined but with tails on
- 1 large egg, beaten
- ½ cup gluten-free bread crumbs
- 1 tablespoon mayonnaise
- ½ teaspoon lemon juice

- 1 teaspoon seasoned salt
- ¼ teaspoon ground black pepper
- ½ pound fresh lump crabmeat, picked over for shells and cartilage
- 2 tablespoons dairy-free buttery spread, melted

Directions :

1. Preheat oven to 375°F. Spray a 9" × 13" baking pan with gluten-free nonstick cooking spray.
2. In a medium skillet, heat olive oil over medium-high heat. Add celery, garlic, and onions and cook for 4 minutes, stirring until softened. Remove from heat and allow to cool.
3. Butterfly each shrimp along the outside curve. Open shrimp flat and place butterflied-side up in prepared baking dish.
4. In a small bowl, combine egg, bread crumbs, mayonnaise, lemon juice, salt, and pepper. Stir in crabmeat.
5. Place 2 tablespoons stuffing onto each shrimp, pressing gently. Drizzle buttery spread over shrimp and bake 20 minutes or until stuffing is golden brown and shrimp are pink.

Lemon Garlic Sautéed Scallops

Ingredients :
- 2 tablespoons olive oil
- 1¼ pounds scallops
- ½ teaspoon salt
- ¼ teaspoon ground black pepper
- 3 tablespoons dairy-free buttery spread, divided
- 2 teaspoons jarred minced garlic
- ¼ cup white wine
- 2 tablespoons lemon juice
- ¼ cup chopped fresh parsley

Directions :

1. Heat olive oil in a large skillet over medium-high heat. Season scallops with salt and pepper. Add scallops in a single layer to the skillet and fry for 1½ minutes on one side until a golden crust forms underneath. Turn over and fry for 1½ minutes until crisp, lightly browned, cooked through, and opaque. Remove from the skillet and transfer to a plate.
2. Melt 2 tablespoons buttery spread in the skillet. Add in garlic and cook 1 minute until fragrant. Pour in wine and bring to a simmer for 2 minutes until wine reduces by half. Stir in the remaining tablespoon buttery spread and lemon juice.
3. Remove the skillet from the heat and add scallops back into the skillet to warm up. Garnish with parsley and serve.

Baked Salmon with Lemon

Ingredients :
- 2 tablespoons olive oil
- 2 teaspoons lemon zest
- 2 tablespoons fresh lemon juice
- 4 (6-ounce) salmon fillets
- ½ teaspoon salt
- ¼ teaspoon ground black pepper
- 1 small lemon, sliced

Directions :

1. Preheat oven to 400°F degrees and grease a 9" × 13" baking dish with gluten-free nonstick cooking spray.

2. In a large bowl, whisk together olive oil, lemon zest, and lemon juice.

3. Place salmon fillets in baking dish. Season tops of salmon with salt and pepper. Drizzle tops evenly with the lemon mixture and gently rub over salmon.

4. Let salmon rest at room temperature for 10 minutes. Place a lemon slice on top of each fillet, then bake 12–16 minutes or until salmon has cooked through.

Cilantro Lime Shrimp Bake

Ingredients :
- 2 pounds raw shrimp, peeled and deveined
- 2 teaspoons jarred minced garlic
- ¼ cup lime juice
- 1 teaspoon ground cumin
- ¼ teaspoon salt
- ¼ teaspoon ground black pepper
- 2 tablespoons dairy-free buttery spread, melted
- ¼ cup gluten-free panko bread crumbs
- ¼ cup chopped fresh cilantro

Directions :

1. Preheat oven to 425°F. Spray a 9" × 13" baking dish with gluten-free nonstick cooking spray.

2. In a medium bowl, add shrimp, garlic, lime juice, cumin, salt, and pepper and toss to combine. Transfer the mixture to prepared baking dish.

3. In a separate medium bowl, stir together melted buttery spread, panko, and cilantro until combined. Sprinkle the panko mixture evenly on top of shrimp.

4. Bake for 15–18 minutes or until shrimp are pink and no longer opaque.

Clams Casino

- **Ingredients :**
- 1 teaspoon olive oil
- ¾ cup finely diced gluten-free bacon
- 1 cup seeded and finely diced red bell pepper
- 2 teaspoons jarred minced garlic
- ⅓ cup white wine
- 1 tablespoon onion powder
- ½ teaspoon salt
- ¼ ground black pepper
- 18 medium (2½") littleneck clams, shucked and bottom shells reserved

Directions :

1. Heat olive oil in a large skillet over medium heat. Add bacon and sauté 3 minutes until crisp. Using a slotted spoon, transfer bacon to a paper towel–lined plate. Add bell peppers and garlic to the skillet and sauté for 5 minutes until peppers are softened. Add wine and simmer for 2 minutes until it is almost evaporated. Remove the skillet from the heat and cool completely. Stir bacon into the vegetable mixture. Season with onion powder, salt, and black pepper.

2. Preheat oven to 500°F. Line a large baking sheet with aluminum foil and spray with gluten-free nonstick cooking spray. Arrange clams in their shells on the baking sheet. Spoon the vegetable mixture atop the clams, dividing equally and mounding slightly. Bake for 10 minutes until topping is golden brown and cooked thoroughly.

New England Clam Bake

- **Ingredients :**
- 1 teaspoon olive oil
- 4 gluten-free chorizo sausages
- 1 cup cold water
- 2 cups white wine
- 3 tablespoons Old Bay Seasoning
- 1 teaspoon salt
- 2 tablespoons jarred minced garlic
- 2 bay leaves
- 2 tablespoons dried thyme
- 1 red onion, peeled and chopped
- 2 pounds new potatoes, halved
- 2 (2-pound) lobsters
- 2 dozen clams
- 4 ears fresh corn, cut into quarters

Directions :

1. In a large stockpot or lobster pot, heat olive oil over medium heat. Pierce sausages in several places with the tip of knife, then add them to the pot with hot oil. Cook for 5 minutes or until golden brown. Transfer to a plate.

2. In the same stockpot, bring the water, wine, Old Bay Seasoning, salt, garlic, bay leaves, and thyme to a boil.

3. Add onions and potatoes, cover, and cook over medium-high heat for 15 minutes. Add lobsters on top, cover, and cook for 3 minutes. Add clams and corn and continue to cook covered for 8–10 minutes until clams open. Carefully remove seafood and vegetables from the pot and transfer to a large platter. Discard bay leaves.

Oven-Fried Orange Roughy

- **Ingredients :**
- ¼ cup gluten-free cornmeal
- ¼ cup gluten-free bread crumbs
- 2 teaspoons seasoned salt
- ½ teaspoon dried dill
- ⅛ teaspoon ground black pepper
- ¼ cup unsweetened almond milk
- 1 pound orange roughy, cut into 1½" × 2" pieces
- 3 tablespoons dairy-free buttery spread, melted

Directions :

1. Preheat oven to 500°F and move oven rack to the position slightly above the middle of oven. Spray a 9" × 13" baking dish with gluten-free nonstick cooking spray.

2. Mix cornmeal, bread crumbs, seasoned salt, dill, and pepper together in a pie pan. Pour milk into a separate pie pan.

3. Dip fish pieces into milk and then press into the bread-crumb mixture to coat on all sides. Place breaded fish into the baking dish. Drizzle buttery spread over breaded fish pieces.

4. Bake for 10 minutes until fish flakes easily with a fork.

Grilled Grouper with Lemon Butter Sauce

- **Ingredients :**
- 4 (8-ounce) grouper fillets, skin removed
- ½ teaspoon salt
- ¼ teaspoon ground black pepper
- 2 tablespoons olive oil

- 1 teaspoon jarred minced garlic
- 1 cup gluten-free chicken broth
- ¼ cup lemon juice
- 2 tablespoons capers, drained and rinsed
- 2 tablespoons dairy-free buttery spread

Directions :

1. Place fillets on an aluminum foil–lined baking sheet sprayed with gluten-free nonstick cooking spray. Salt and pepper fillets. Broil 4" from the heat for 6–7 minutes on each side or until fish flakes easily with a fork. Remove from oven.

2. Heat olive oil in a medium skillet over medium heat. Add garlic and cook for 30 seconds until fragrant. Pour in broth and lemon juice and bring the mixture to a boil. Boil for 5–8 minutes, stirring occasionally, until sauce reduces. Add capers and buttery spread to the pan and stir to combine; cook 2–3 minutes until buttery spread is melted.

3. Serve with sauce poured over fillets.

Pecan-Crusted Honey Mustard Salmon

- **Ingredients :**
- 4 (4-ounce) salmon fillets
- ½ teaspoon salt
- ¼ teaspoon ground black pepper
- 2 tablespoons stone-ground mustard
- 2 tablespoons honey
- ½ teaspoon paprika
- ½ cup pecans

Directions :

1. Preheat oven to 375°F. Line a baking sheet with aluminum foil and spray with gluten-free nonstick cooking spray.

2. Place salmon fillets on prepared baking sheet skin-side down and sprinkle with salt and pepper.

3. In a small bowl, mix mustard and honey. Pour the mixture over each salmon piece and rub the mixture into salmon on all sides.

4. Add pecans to a food processor and finely chop. Stir paprika into pecans. Evenly distribute the pecan mixture on top of each salmon fillet. Press the mixture into salmon to create a crust. Bake for 9–13 minutes.

Chili Lime Tilapia with Fresh Mango Salsa

Ingredients :

MANGO SALSA
- 1 small mango, peeled, pitted, and diced
- 2 tablespoons seeded and finely diced red bell pepper
- 2 tablespoons peeled and finely diced red onion
- ½ cup chopped fresh cilantro
- 1 tablespoon seeded and finely chopped jalapeño
- ¼ cup lime juice
- ¼ teaspoon salt

TILAPIA
- 2 teaspoons chili powder
- 1 teaspoon garlic powder
- 1 teaspoon onion powder
- ¾ teaspoon salt
- 1 teaspoon light brown sugar, packed
- ¼ cup lime juice
- ¼ cup olive oil
- 4 (6-ounce) tilapia fillets

Directions :

1. In a medium bowl, combine the mango, bell peppers, onions, cilantro, and jalapeño. Add lime juice and salt and mix well. Cover and refrigerate for at least 1 hour.

2. Preheat oven to 350°F. Line a baking sheet with aluminum foil and spray with gluten-free nonstick cooking spray.

3. In a small bowl, whisk together chili powder, garlic powder, onion powder, salt, brown sugar, lime juice, and olive oil.

4. Pat tilapia fillets dry with a paper towel and place on prepared baking sheet. Pour sauce over fish and bake for 15–20 minutes. When finished, plate and top with mango salsa.

Marinated Grilled Tuna Steaks

- **Ingredients :**
- 8 tablespoons olive oil, divided
- 4 teaspoons Old Bay Seasoning
- 1 tablespoon lime juice
- 1 tablespoon lemon juice
- 4 (6-ounce, 1"-thick) fresh tuna steaks

Directions :

1. In a large bowl, combine 4 tablespoons of olive oil, Old Bay Seasoning, lime juice, and lemon juice.

2. Add tuna steaks to the bowl. Cover and place in the refrigerator for 20 minutes, turning tuna occasionally.

3. Add 2 tablespoons oil to a stove-top cast-iron grill and heat over high heat. Brush tuna with 2 tablespoons of oil. Grill tuna on each side for 2–2½ minutes. The center should be bright pink. Allow tuna to rest for 5–10 minutes before serving.

Greek-Style Snapper

- **Ingredients :**
- 1 tablespoon olive oil
- 1 small sweet onion, peeled and chopped
- 1 tablespoon jarred minced garlic
- 1 (14.5-ounce) can diced tomatoes, drained
- ½ cup gluten-free chicken broth
- 1 tablespoon red wine vinegar
- 2 tablespoons lemon juice
- ⅓ cup sliced Kalamata olives
- 1 teaspoon dried oregano
- 1 teaspoon dried dill
- 1 pound red snapper fillet
- 2 tablespoons chopped fresh parsley

Directions :

1. Preheat oven to 425°F. Spray a 9" × 13" baking dish with gluten-free nonstick cooking spray.

2. Heat olive oil in a large skillet over medium-high heat. Sauté onions and garlic for 2 minutes. Stir in tomatoes, broth, vinegar, lemon juice, olives, oregano, and dill; simmer for 5 minutes.

3. Place fillets in prepared baking dish. Spoon tomato mixture over fillets. Bake for 10–15 minutes until fish flakes with a fork. Remove from oven, plate, and sprinkle with parsley.

New Orleans–Style Barbecue Shrimp

- **Ingredients :**
- 1 cup dairy-free buttery spread
- ¼ cup lemon juice
- 2 tablespoons gluten-free Worcestershire sauce
- 1 tablespoon jarred minced garlic
- 1 tablespoon onion powder
- 1 teaspoon dried oregano
- 1 teaspoon dried thyme
- 1 teaspoon dried basil

- 1 teaspoon paprika
- ¼ teaspoon cayenne pepper
- 2 teaspoons salt
- ½ teaspoon ground black pepper
- 2 pounds large shrimp, not peeled

Directions:

1. In a large skillet, melt the buttery spread over medium-high heat. Reduce the heat to medium-low and add lemon juice, Worcestershire sauce, garlic, onion powder, oregano, thyme, basil, paprika, cayenne pepper, salt, and black pepper. Stir and simmer for about 5 minutes.

2. Add shrimp and increase the heat to medium. Cook for 4–5 minutes, occasionally turning shrimp, until shrimp to turn pink. Cover the skillet and remove it from the heat. Let sit for 15 minutes, stirring every 5 minutes. Serve.

Spaghetti with White Clam Sauce

Ingredients:
- 1 (12-ounce) package gluten-free spaghetti
- 3 tablespoons olive oil
- 2 tablespoons jarred minced garlic
- 1 teaspoon dried thyme
- ¼ teaspoon crushed red pepper flakes
- ½ cup white wine
- 1 (15-ounce) can whole baby clams in juice
- ¼ teaspoon salt
- ¼ cup chopped fresh parsley

Directions:

1. Cook pasta to al dente according to the package directions.

2. Add olive oil to a large skillet and heat over medium heat. Add garlic, thyme, and red pepper flakes and sauté for 1 minute. Add wine to the skillet and stir. Stir in clams and their juice. Add pasta to clam sauce. Toss and coat pasta in sauce and cook for 2–3 minutes. Remove from heat and season with salt and parsley and serve.

Curried Shrimp

Ingredients:
- 2 tablespoons olive oil
- ½ large yellow onion, peeled and diced
- 2 tablespoons jarred minced garlic
- 2 tablespoons jarred minced ginger

- 1 (15-ounce) can unsweetened coconut milk
- 2 tablespoons curry powder
- ½ teaspoon ground cumin
- ⅛ teaspoon ground cinnamon
- ¼ cup lime juice
- ¼ teaspoon salt
- ⅛ teaspoon ground black pepper
- 1½ pounds raw shrimp, peeled and deveined
- ½ cup chopped fresh cilantro

Directions :

1. In a large skillet, heat olive oil over medium-high heat. Add onions, garlic, and ginger to the skillet and sauté for 2–4 minutes. Add in milk, curry powder, cumin, cinnamon, lime juice, salt, and pepper and stir to combine. Bring to a boil, then reduce heat to medium-low and let simmer for 7–10 minutes.

2. Add in shrimp and let simmer for an additional 5–7 minutes until shrimp is cooked through. Top with cilantro.

Crispy Baked Fish Sticks

Ingredients :
- 1 pound cod fillets, cut into 1" strips
- 2 teaspoons seasoned salt
- 1 cup gluten-free all-purpose flour with xanthan gum
- 2 large eggs
- 1 tablespoon Dijon mustard
- 1 cup gluten-free panko bread crumbs
- 1 cup gluten-free bread crumbs
- ½ teaspoon garlic powder
- ½ teaspoon onion powder

Directions :

1. Preheat oven to 400°F and line a baking sheet with aluminum foil and spray with gluten-free nonstick cooking spray.

2. Season fish with seasoned salt. Add flour to a pie pan or shallow dish. In a second pie pan, whisk together eggs and mustard. In a third pie pan, combine panko, bread crumbs, garlic powder, and onion powder.

3. Press a fish stick in flour, making sure to cover all sides. Next dredge fish stick in the egg mixture. Then press fish stick in the bread-crumb mixture, patting to help coating adhere. Place coated fish stick on prepared baking sheet and repeat the process with remaining fish sticks. Spray fish with olive oil gluten-free nonstick cooking spray.

4. Bake for 6 minutes, then turn over fish sticks and spray with cooking spray again. Bake another 6–10 minutes until fish begins to flake easily with a fork.

Roasted Garlic Potatoes

- **Ingredients :**
- ¼ cup olive oil
- 2 teaspoons salt
- ¼ teaspoon ground black pepper
- 2 tablespoons jarred minced garlic
- 3 pounds small red potatoes, cut in half

Directions :

1. Preheat oven to 400°F. Line a baking sheet with aluminum foil and spray with gluten-free nonstick cooking spray.

2. Add olive oil, salt, pepper, and garlic in a large bowl and whisk together. Add potatoes and toss until potatoes are well coated.

3. Place potatoes on prepared sheet and spread out into one layer. Roast in the oven for 45 minutes to 1 hour until browned and crisp.

Easy Rice Pilaf

Ingredients :
- 2 teaspoons olive oil
- ½ cup peeled and chopped sweet onion
- 1 cup uncooked long-grain white rice
- 2 cups gluten-free chicken broth
- 2 teaspoons seasoned salt
- ⅛ teaspoon ground black pepper
- 1 cup frozen peas and carrots

Directions :

1. Heat olive oil in a large skillet over medium heat. Add onions and cook for 3 minutes until translucent. Add rice and stir until rice is lightly toasted.

2. Stir in broth, salt, and pepper and bring to a boil. Reduce heat to a simmer, cover, and cook for 10 minutes.

3. Stir in peas and carrots, cover, and cook for an additional 10 minutes. Fluff with a fork and serve.

Baked Sweet Potato Fries

Ingredients :
- 1 pound sweet potatoes, peeled and cut into ¼" strips
- 2 tablespoons olive oil
- 2 tablespoons cornstarch
- ¼ teaspoon garlic powder
- ½ teaspoon paprika
- ¼ teaspoon ground black pepper
- 1 teaspoon salt

Directions :

1. Add cut potatoes to a large bowl of water and soak for 30 minutes.
2. Preheat oven to 425°F. Line a large baking sheet with parchment paper and spray with gluten-free nonstick cooking spray.
3. Drain potatoes and blot dry with a paper towel. Add potatoes in a separate large bowl. Drizzle evenly with olive oil and toss until potatoes are evenly coated.
4. In a small bowl, whisk together cornstarch, garlic powder, paprika, and pepper until combined. Sprinkle the mixture evenly over potatoes and toss until they are evenly coated and cornstarch has soaked into oil.
5. Spread potatoes out in an even layer on prepared baking sheet, making sure not to overlap. Bake for 25 minutes. Then remove pan from oven and take the time to flip each fry with a spatula. Rearrange so that fries are evenly spaced and not overlapping again. Put back in the oven and bake for 20 minutes. Sprinkle with salt, then allow fries cool for 5 minutes. Serve warm.

Balsamic-Roasted Brussels Sprouts

- **Ingredients :**
- ¼ cup olive oil
- 1 teaspoon salt
- ¼ teaspoon ground black pepper
- 1½ pounds Brussels sprouts, trimmed and cut in half through the core
- 1 tablespoon balsamic vinegar
- 2 tablespoons honey

Directions :

1. Preheat oven to 400°F. Line a baking sheet with aluminum foil and spray with gluten-free nonstick cooking spray.
2. Add olive oil, salt, and pepper to a large bowl and stir to combine. Add Brussels sprouts to the bowl and toss to coat with the oil mixture.
3. Place Brussels sprouts on the baking sheet and roast for 20–30 minutes until tender and browned.

Remove from the oven.

4. Add vinegar and honey to the large bowl and whisk to combine. Add the roasted sprouts to the bowl and toss to cover in the vinegar mixture. Serve warm.

Ratatouille

Ingredients :
- 6 tablespoons olive oil, divided
- 1 large eggplant, cut into ⅓" cubes
- 1 teaspoon salt, divided
- 2 medium zucchini, cut into cubes
- 1 medium yellow onion, peeled and finely chopped
- 1 large red bell pepper, seeded and chopped
- 2 tablespoons jarred minced garlic
- 5 Roma tomatoes, chopped
- 1 tablespoon tomato paste
- 1 tablespoon dried thyme
- 3 tablespoons dried basil
- 1 teaspoon granulated sugar

Directions :

1. In a large skillet, heat 3 tablespoons olive oil over medium heat. Add eggplant and sprinkle with ¼ teaspoon salt. Cook for 10–12 minutes, stirring frequently, until soft and starting to brown. Transfer to a plate.

2. Add 1 more tablespoon olive oil to the skillet and add the zucchini. Cook for 3–4 minutes, stirring frequently, until soft. Season with ¼ teaspoon salt and transfer to a plate.

3. Add remaining 2 tablespoons olive oil to the skillet and add onions, bell peppers, and garlic. Cook for 5 minutes, stirring frequently. Add tomatoes and their juices, tomato paste, thyme, basil, sugar, and remaining ½ teaspoon salt. Cook for 10 minutes, stirring occasionally, until tomatoes are broken down into a sauce.

4. Add eggplant back to the skillet; bring to a gentle boil, then reduce the heat to low and simmer uncovered for about 10 minutes until eggplant is soft. Add zucchini back and cook for 1–2 minutes. Serve warm or chilled.

Creamy Scalloped Potatoes

Ingredients :
- 6 large russet potatoes, peeled and thinly sliced
- 6 tablespoons dairy-free buttery spread
- 4 tablespoons gluten-free flour with xanthan gum

- 1 tablespoon onion powder
- 1 tablespoon garlic powder
- 1 cup gluten-free chicken broth
- 2 cups unsweetened almond milk
- 2 teaspoons salt
- ¼ teaspoon ground black pepper
- 1 teaspoon tarragon

Directions :

1. Preheat oven to 425°F. Lightly grease a 9" × 13" baking pan with gluten-free nonstick cooking spray. Place potato slices in a large bowl of cold water.

2. Melt buttery spread in a medium skillet over medium heat. Whisk in flour. Add onion powder and garlic powder. Pour in broth and whisk until combined. Add in milk, salt, pepper, and tarragon and whisk until combined. Cook for 2 minutes until sauce begins to simmer and thicken. Remove from heat.

3. Drain potato slices. Spread one-third of potato slices into the bottom of prepared baking dish. Top evenly with one-third of cream sauce. Add another layer of potatoes and sauce, and repeat once more for a total of three layers.

4. Bake for 45 minutes until potatoes are cooked through. The sauce should be bubbly around the edges. For a crisp topping, change the oven setting to broil for 5 minutes before removing the dish.

Potato Pancakes

Ingredients :
- 1 large egg
- ¼ cup gluten-free all-purpose flour with xanthan gum
- 2 teaspoons onion powder
- ¼ teaspoon salt
- ⅛ teaspoon ground black pepper
- 2 cups cooked mashed potatoes
- 3 tablespoons vegetable oil

Directions :

1. In a large bowl, whisk together egg, flour, and seasonings. Add the mashed potatoes and stir to combine.

2. Heat oil in a large skillet over medium-high heat. Use an ice cream scoop to drop batter on the skillet. Cook for 5–6 minutes until pancakes start to turn golden brown. Turn pancakes over and press patties down, cooking for another 5–6 minutes, until golden brown.

Honey-Glazed Carrots

Ingredients :
- 1 pound baby carrots
- 2 tablespoons dairy-free buttery spread
- 2 tablespoons honey
- 1 tablespoon lemon juice
- ¼ teaspoon salt
- 2 teaspoons dried dill

Directions :

1. In a medium saucepan, bring water to a boil over medium-high heat. Add carrots and cook 10–15 minutes until tender. Drain carrots and add back to the pan with buttery spread, honey, and lemon juice and stir to combine ingredients.

2. Cook for 5 minutes until glaze coats carrots. Season with salt and dill.

Southwestern Black Bean and Corn Salad

Ingredients :
- 1 tablespoon olive oil
- ½ cup lime juice
- ¼ teaspoon gluten-free and dairy-free hot sauce
- ½ teaspoon salt
- 1 (15-ounce) can black beans, rinsed and drained
- 1 (15-ounce) can corn, drained
- 1 large tomato, chopped
- ⅓ cup peeled and chopped red onion
- 1 cup chopped fresh cilantro

Directions :

1. Whisk together olive oil, lime juice, hot sauce, and salt in a small bowl.

2. In a large bowl, combine beans, corn, tomatoes, onions, and cilantro. Pour lime dressing over salad ingredients to coat. Cover and refrigerate for 30 minutes before serving.

Cheesy Green Bean Casserole

Ingredients :
- 2 (14-ounce) cans French-style green beans, drained
- 1 teaspoon onion powder
- 1 cup gluten-free and dairy-free Cream of Mushroom Soup
- 1½ cups shredded dairy-free Cheddar cheese
- 1 cup crushed gluten-free potato sticks

Directions :

1. Preheat oven to 350°F. Spray a 2-quart casserole dish with gluten-free nonstick cooking spray.
2. Add beans to prepared dish. Sprinkle onion powder over beans. Pour soup over the bean mixture and stir to combine. Add cheese and stir to combine.
3. Bake on the middle rack for 15 minutes. Add potato sticks and bake for an additional 15–25 minutes or until sides are bubbly and potato sticks are golden brown.

Italian Roasted Vegetables

Ingredients :
- 1 large zucchini, sliced
- 1 large yellow squash, sliced
- 2 large russet potatoes, diced
- 1 cup halved grape tomatoes
- 2 tablespoons olive oil
- 1 teaspoon salt
- 2 tablespoons dried basil

Directions :
1. Preheat oven to 425°F. Line a baking sheet with aluminum foil and spray with gluten-free nonstick cooking spray.
2. In a large bowl, toss all vegetables together with olive oil, salt, and basil.
3. Place vegetables on prepared baking sheet. Bake for 35–40 minutes.

Roasted Butternut Squash

Ingredients :
- 3 tablespoons olive oil
- ½ teaspoon salt
- ⅛ teaspoon ground black pepper
- 1 large butternut squash, peeled, seeded, and cut into 1" cubes

Directions :
1. Preheat oven to 400°F. Line a baking sheet with aluminum foil and spray with gluten-free nonstick cooking spray.
2. Add olive oil, salt, and pepper to a large bowl and stir to combine. Add squash and toss.
3. Place squash on prepared sheet and arrange squash in one layer. Bake for 25–30 minutes until the squash is tender and starting to brown on the edges.

Sautéed Garlic Green Beans

Ingredients :
- 1 pound green beans, trimmed
- 1 teaspoon salt, divided
- 2 tablespoons olive oil
- 1 tablespoon jarred minced garlic

Directions :

1. Bring a large pot of water to a boil over medium-high heat. Add beans and ½ teaspoon salt and cook for 4 minutes. Drain beans in a colander.

2. Heat olive oil in a large skillet over medium-high heat. Add garlic and sauté for 30 seconds until fragrant. Add green beans and toss to coat with the oil mixture. Sauté beans for 2–4 minutes until they get a little caramelization. Add remaining salt and serve warm.

Zucchini Noodles

Ingredients :
- 4 medium zucchini, spiralized
- ½ teaspoon salt
- 1 tablespoon olive oil

Directions :

1. Place zoodles in a colander, toss them with salt, and let sit for 20 minutes. Squeeze out excess water from zoodles with a paper towel.

2. Add olive oil to a large skillet and heat over medium-high heat. Add zucchini to the skillet and sauté for 3–5 minutes.

Easy Oven-Roasted Corn on the Cob

Ingredients :
- 6 ears of corn, in husks
- ½ teaspoon salt
- ¼ cup dairy-free buttery spread, melted

Directions :

1. Preheat oven to 375°F.

2. Place ears of corn with the husks still on them on an ungreased baking sheet. Bake for 40 minutes.

3. Remove from the oven and allow to cool for several minutes. Peel back corn husks and snap the ends off. Serve with salt and buttery spread.

Southern-Style Sweet Potato Casserole

Ingredients :
- 3 cups cooked sweet potatoes
- ⅓ cup dairy-free buttery spread, melted
- 1 cup granulated sugar
- ⅛ teaspoon ground ginger
- 2 teaspoons ground cinnamon
- ¼ teaspoon ground nutmeg
- 2 large eggs
- 1 teaspoon pure vanilla extract
- ¼ cup unsweetened almond milk
- 3 cups gluten-free mini marshmallows

Directions :

1. Preheat oven to 350°F and spray a 2-quart casserole dish with gluten-free nonstick cooking spray.

2. In a large bowl, beat mashed sweet potatoes, buttery spread, sugar, ginger, cinnamon, nutmeg, eggs, vanilla, and milk with an electric mixer until smooth. Pour the sweet potato mixture into prepared dish.

3. Bake for 30 minutes. Remove from the oven and top with mini marshmallows and bake for an additional 5–10 minutes. Watch the marshmallows carefully because all ovens are different—be sure they do not burn.

Bacon and Tomato Macaroni Salad

Ingredients :
- 1 (12-ounce) box gluten-free elbow macaroni noodles, cooked
- 1 cup mayonnaise
- 2 tablespoons white vinegar
- 1 tablespoon yellow mustard
- ⅔ cup sugar
- 1½ teaspoons salt
- ½ teaspoon ground black pepper
- 1 teaspoon onion powder
- 1 cup chopped cooked gluten-free bacon
- 1 cup quartered grape tomatoes

Directions :

1. Cook macaroni according to the package directions for al dente. After draining the pasta, rinse pasta with cold water. Add pasta to a large bowl.

2. In a small bowl, add mayonnaise, vinegar, mustard, sugar, salt, pepper, and onion powder and stir

until fully combined. Add to pasta and stir until fully coated.

3. Add bacon and tomatoes to pasta and stir until fully combined. Cover and refrigerate for 30 minutes before serving.

Loaded Bacon Ranch Potato Salad

Ingredients :
- 4 cups diced russet potatoes
- 1 tablespoon dried dill
- 1½ teaspoons garlic powder
- 1½ teaspoons onion powder
- 2 teaspoons dried parsley
- 1½ teaspoons salt
- ½ teaspoon ground black pepper
- 1 tablespoon granulated sugar
- 1 cup mayonnaise
- 1¼ cups chopped cooked gluten-free bacon, divided
- ½ cup sliced green onion, divided
- 2 large hard-boiled eggs, chopped

Directions :

1. Add potatoes to a large pot and cover with water. Cook over high heat and bring to a boil. Once boiling, reduce the heat to medium and boil for 12–15 minutes or until potatoes are tender. Check with a fork to see if potatoes are cooked to your liking.

2. Drain potatoes and rinse with cold water. Add potatoes to a large bowl and place in the refrigerator to cool while you are making the dressing.

3. In a small bowl, add all seasonings and sugar together and stir to combine. Add mayonnaise and mix until fully combined.

4. Add dressing to chilled potatoes. Carefully stir to fully cover potatoes with dressing.

5. Add 1 cup bacon, ¼ cup green onions, and eggs to potato salad. Stir gently. Cover and chill for 2 hours. Sprinkle remaining ¼ cup of the bacon and remaining ¼ cup green onions on top of potato salad before serving.

Savory Stuffing

Ingredients :
- 1 tablespoon olive oil
- 1 cup diced celery

- ½ teaspoon jarred minced garlic
- 1 teaspoon salt
- 1 tablespoon onion powder
- 1 tablespoon dried thyme
- 1 tablespoon dried sage
- 1 teaspoon dried rosemary
- 1 loaf gluten-free and dairy-free sandwich bread, cut into 1" cubes
- 2 large eggs, whisked
- 2 cups gluten-free chicken broth

Directions :

1. Preheat oven to 350°F and spray a 2½-quart casserole dish with gluten-free nonstick cooking spray.

2. Add olive oil, celery, and jarred minced garlic to a small skillet and sauté over medium-high heat until soft, about 8–10 minutes.

3. Add spices to a small bowl and stir to combine.

4. Add bread pieces to a large bowl. Pour seasoning blend and whisked eggs over bread and stir. Add the celery mixture and stir. Add chicken broth and gently mix until bread is evenly moistened.

5. Pour the stuffing mixture into prepared dish.

6. Bake for 40–50 minutes until the top of stuffing is golden brown and lightly crisp.

Easy Homemade Gravy

Ingredients :
- 2 cups gluten-free chicken broth
- 3 tablespoons water
- 3 tablespoons cornstarch
- ¼ teaspoon salt
- ⅛ teaspoon pepper

Directions :

1. Add broth to a small saucepan over medium heat. Whisk water and cornstarch in a small bowl until smooth and add to broth, stirring constantly with a whisk, bringing to a boil.

2. Boil for 1 minute and season with salt and pepper. Serve warm.

Creamy Dill Sauce

Ingredients :
- ½ cup mayonnaise
- 1 tablespoon dried dill
- 1 teaspoon horseradish sauce

- 1 teaspoon lemon juice
- ¼ teaspoon garlic salt

Directions :

1. Combine all ingredients in a small bowl. Cover and chill in the refrigerator for 30 minutes before serving. Store in an airtight container in the refrigerator for up to Directions week.

Homemade Buttermilk Ranch Dressing

- **Ingredients :**
- 1 cup unsweetened almond milk
- 1 tablespoon white vinegar
- ½ cup mayonnaise
- 1 tablespoon dried dill
- 1½ teaspoons garlic powder
- 1½ teaspoons onion powder
- 2 teaspoons dried parsley
- 1½ teaspoons salt
- ½ teaspoon ground black pepper
- 1 tablespoon granulated sugar

Directions :

1. Add milk and vinegar to a small bowl and place in the refrigerator for 5–10 minutes to make buttermilk.
2. In a separate small bowl, add mayonnaise, seasonings, and sugar and whisk together. Pour in buttermilk and whisk. Cover and refrigerate for 30 minutes before stirring again and serving.

Homemade Honey Mustard Dressing

Ingredients :
- ½ cup mayonnaise
- 2 tablespoons Dijon mustard
- 2 tablespoons honey
- 4 teaspoons lemon juice

Directions :

1. In a small bowl, whisk together all ingredients. Cover and refrigerate for 30 minutes before serving. Stir well before serving.

Balsamic Vinaigrette Salad Dressing

Ingredients :
- ½ teaspoon dried basil
- ½ teaspoon garlic powder
- ½ teaspoon onion powder
- ½ teaspoon dried oregano
- 1 teaspoon salt
- 2 tablespoons honey
- 2 tablespoons water
- ⅓ cup vinegar blend (made up of half apple cider vinegar, and half balsamic vinegar)
- ⅔ cup olive oil

Directions :

1. In a small bowl, mix seasonings together.
2. Add honey, water, vinegar blend, and olive oil to dry ingredients and whisk until all ingredients are fully combined.
3. Cover and refrigerate for 30 minutes before serving. Stir well before serving.

Homemade Tartar Sauce

- **Ingredients :**
- 1 cup mayonnaise
- 1 cup finely chopped dill pickles
- 2 tablespoons peeled and finely chopped sweet onion
- 1 tablespoon dried dill
- 1 tablespoon lemon juice
- 1 teaspoon granulated sugar
- ⅛ teaspoon freshly ground black pepper

Directions :

1. In a small bowl, whisk together all ingredients. Cover and refrigerate for 30 minutes before serving. Stir before serving.

Bread Machine Bread

Ingredients :
- 1½ cups unsweetened almond milk, warm
- ¼ cup dairy-free buttery spread, melted
- ½ cup honey
- 2 large eggs, room temperature and whisked
- 1 teaspoon apple cider vinegar
- 3 cups gluten-free all-purpose flour with xanthan gum

- 1 teaspoon salt
- 1¾ teaspoons instant yeast

Directions :

1. Grease a bread pan with gluten-free nonstick cooking spray.
2. Pour warm milk, buttery spread, honey, eggs, and vinegar into the bread pan.
3. Add flour and salt to the bread pan. Make a small hole with your finger in the flour. Pour yeast into the hole.
4. Start the bread machine and set to the gluten-free setting. As bread machine is mixing, you may need to go in and scrape the sides down into the batter with a spatula.
5. Once the bread machine has finished the baking cycle, allow bread to cool 5–10 minutes before removing from the pan and slicing. Store in an airtight container at room temperature for up to 3 days.

Easy One-Bowl Banana Bread

- **Ingredients :**
- 2 large ripe bananas, peeled
- 1 teaspoon baking soda
- ⅓ cup dairy-free buttery spread, melted
- ⅛ teaspoon salt
- ¾ cup granulated sugar
- 2 large eggs, whisked
- 1 teaspoon pure vanilla extract
- 1½ cups gluten-free all-purpose flour with xanthan gum

Directions :

1. Preheat oven to 350°F. Spray a 4" × 8" loaf pan with gluten-free nonstick cooking spray.
2. In a large bowl, mash bananas until smooth, add baking soda, and stir to combine. Add buttery spread. Stir in salt, sugar, eggs, and vanilla extract. Mix in flour. Pour batter into prepared loaf pan.
3. Bake on the center rack for 50 minutes to 1 hour or until a toothpick inserted in the center comes out clean. Allow bread to cool for 3–5 minutes before removing from the pan for further cooling and slicing.

Double Chocolate Banana Bread

Ingredients :
- 2 ripe large bananas, peeled and mashed
- 1 teaspoon baking soda
- ⅓ cup dairy-free buttery spread, melted

- ¾ cup sugar
- ¼ cup cocoa powder
- ⅛ teaspoon salt
- 2 large eggs, whisked
- 1 teaspoon pure vanilla extract
- 1½ cups gluten-free all-purpose flour with xanthan gum
- ½ cup gluten-free and dairy-free mini chocolate chips

Directions :

1. Preheat oven to 350°F. Spray a 4" × 8" loaf pan with gluten-free nonstick cooking spray.

2. In a large bowl, combine bananas and baking soda. Stir in buttery spread, sugar, cocoa powder, salt, eggs, and vanilla. Mix in flour. Stir in chocolate chips. Pour batter into prepared loaf pan.

3. Bake on the center rack for 50 minutes to 1 hour or until a toothpick inserted in the center comes out clean. Allow bread to cool for 3–5 minutes before removing from the pan and slicing. Store leftovers in an airtight container at room temperature for up to 3 days.

Soft Homemade Dinner Rolls

Ingredients :
- 3 cups gluten-free all-purpose flour with xanthan gum
- 1 teaspoon salt
- 1¾ teaspoons instant yeast
- 1¼ cups unsweetened almond milk, warmed to 110°F–115°F
- ¼ cup dairy-free buttery spread, softened
- 2 large eggs, room temperature
- 1 teaspoon apple cider vinegar
- ½ cup honey
- 2 tablespoons dairy-free buttery spread, melted

Directions :

1. Preheat oven to 200°F. Once it gets to 100°F, turn off oven. Spray two 9" metal cake pans with gluten-free nonstick cooking spray.

2. In a large bowl, add flour and salt. Make a small hole in the center and pour yeast into the hole.

3. Check the temperature of warm milk with a thermometer. (If your milk is too hot it will kill the yeast.) Pour milk over yeast.

4. Add softened buttery spread, eggs, vinegar, and honey to the flour mixture and mix for 2–3 minutes until fully combined. The dough will be sticky.

5. Using a greased ice cream scoop, scoop dough balls and place into prepared pans. Take a small spatula and smooth out the tops of dough. There will be eight dough balls around each pan and one

dough ball in the center. Cover the pans with a kitchen towel and allow to rise in the warm oven for 1 hour. Take the pans out and keep covered while preheating the oven.

6. Preheat oven to 400°F. Bake rolls on the middle rack for 14–16 minutes until light golden brown. The temperature of the rolls should measure 200°F internally. Melt 2 tablespoons buttery spread in a small microwave-safe bowl and brush the tops of rolls before serving warm.

Easy Thick-Crust Pizza Dough

- **Ingredients :**
- 2½ cups plus 2 tablespoons gluten-free all-purpose flour with xanthan gum, divided
- 1 packet (2¼ teaspoons) instant yeast
- 1 tablespoon gluten-free baking powder
- 1 teaspoon salt
- 1 tablespoon honey
- 1½ cups warm water (110°F–115°F)
- ½ cup olive oil
- 1 teaspoon apple cider vinegar

Directions :

1. Preheat oven to 200°F. Once it gets to 100°F, turn off oven.

2. In a large bowl, combine 2½ cups flour, yeast, baking powder, and salt.

3. In a small bowl, add honey and warm water and stir until honey is dissolved.

4. Pour the honey mixture into the flour mixture and mix with your mixer with a dough hook or paddle attachment on low.

5. Pour olive oil and vinegar into the dough mixture and mix on medium speed for 3 minutes. The dough will be very sticky.

6. Place dough in a large ovenproof bowl sprayed with gluten-free nonstick cooking spray. Cover with plastic wrap and then with a kitchen towel and place in warm oven for 30 minutes to rise.

7. Remove dough from the oven and preheat oven to 425°F.

8. Pour remaining 2 tablespoons flour onto a sheet of parchment paper and spread into a large 15" circle.

9. Turn the bowl over on top of floured parchment paper. Gently pat dough into a circle in an outward motion. Work from the middle and push to spread the dough out to the edge to make a 15" circle. Use your fingertips to press down into the dough to form the crust edge. Use your hands to finish shaping and rounding the edges.

10. Place the parchment paper on a pizza pan or baking sheet. Bake for 15 minutes. Remove the pizza crust from the oven and top with your favorite toppings. Bake for another 5 minutes, until the crust is golden brown. Allow the pizza to cool for 2–3 minutes before slicing.

Chocolate Chip Quick Bread

Ingredients :
- ⅓ cup dairy-free buttery spread, melted
- 2 large eggs, whisked
- 1 tablespoon pure vanilla extract
- 1½ cups gluten-free all-purpose flour with xanthan gum
- ½ cup sugar
- 1 teaspoon baking soda
- ½ teaspoon gluten-free baking powder
- ¼ teaspoon salt
- 1 cup unsweetened almond milk
- 1 cup gluten-free and dairy-free chocolate chips

Directions :

1. Preheat oven to 350°F. Spray a 4" × 8" loaf pan with gluten-free nonstick cooking spray.

2. In a large bowl, add buttery spread, eggs, and vanilla and stir to combine. Add flour, sugar, baking soda, baking powder, and salt and mix until fully combined. Add milk and mix until smooth. Stir in chocolate chips.

3. Pour batter into a prepared loaf pan. Bake on the center rack for 50 minutes to 1 hour or until a toothpick inserted in the center comes out clean. Allow bread to cool for 3–5 minutes before removing from the pan and slicing. Store leftovers in an airtight container at room temperature for up to 3 days.

Southern Sweet Corn Bread

Ingredients :
- 1½ cups unsweetened almond milk
- 1½ tablespoons white vinegar
- 1½ cups gluten-free cornmeal
- 1 cup gluten-free all-purpose flour with xanthan gum
- ½ cup sugar
- ½ teaspoon baking soda
- 2 teaspoons gluten-free baking powder
- 1 teaspoon salt
- ½ cup dairy-free buttery spread, melted
- 1 tablespoon honey
- 2 large eggs, whisked

Directions :

1. Preheat oven to 400°F. Spray the bottom and sides of an 8" square pan or 8" cast-iron pan with gluten-free nonstick cooking spray.

2. In a small bowl, add milk and vinegar together and allow to sit for 2 minutes to make buttermilk.

3. In a large bowl, mix together cornmeal, flour, sugar, baking soda, baking powder, and salt.

4. Stir in buttery spread, honey, eggs, and the milk mixture and mix until fully combined.

5. Pour batter into prepared pan and smooth top of batter. Bake 20–25 minutes or until golden brown and a toothpick inserted in the center comes out clean. Cool for 5 minutes before cutting. Serve warm.

Apple Cinnamon Quick Bread

Ingredients :
- 1½ cups applesauce
- ⅓ cup dairy-free buttery spread, melted
- ½ cup sugar
- 2 large eggs, whisked
- 1 teaspoon pure vanilla extract
- 1½ cups gluten-free all-purpose flour with xanthan gum
- 1 teaspoon baking soda
- ½ teaspoon gluten-free baking powder
- 1 tablespoon ground cinnamon
- ⅛ teaspoon salt
- 1 cup unsweetened almond milk

Directions :

1. Preheat oven to 350°F. Spray a 4" × 8" loaf pan with gluten-free nonstick cooking spray.

2. Add applesauce to a large bowl. Stir in buttery spread, sugar, eggs, and vanilla extract. Mix in flour, baking soda, baking powder, cinnamon, and salt and mix until all ingredients are fully combined. Add milk and mix until smooth. Pour batter into prepared loaf pan.

3. Bake on the center rack for 50 minutes to 1 hour or until a toothpick inserted in the center comes out clean. Allow the bread to cool for 3–5 minutes before removing from the pan and slicing. Store leftovers in an airtight container at room temperature for up to 3 days.

Southern Buttermilk Biscuits

Ingredients :
- 8 tablespoons dairy-free buttery spread, divided
- 1 cup unsweetened almond milk
- 1 tablespoon white vinegar
- 2 cups plus 2 tablespoons gluten-free all-purpose flour with xanthan gum, divided

- 1 tablespoon gluten-free baking powder
- 1 teaspoon salt
- 2 tablespoons granulated sugar
- 1 large egg, whisked

Directions :

1. Preheat oven to 450°F and grease a large cast-iron pan with vegetable oil or line a baking sheet with parchment paper.

2. Add 6 tablespoons buttery spread in a small bowl and place in the freezer for 5 minutes. In a separate small bowl, add milk and vinegar, then let stand 5 minutes in the refrigerator to keep cold.

3. In a large bowl, stir together 2 cups flour, baking powder, salt, and sugar.

4. Cut in chilled buttery spread into flour with a pastry cutter or fork until it looks like small peas.

5. Add in the milk mixture and whisked egg and stir until a soft dough forms. The key is to not overmix because that will create tough biscuits. The dough will be sticky.

6. Add 1 tablespoon flour to a large piece of parchment paper. Place dough on top of floured parchment paper. Dust the top of dough with remaining 1 tablespoon flour and gently fold dough in half on top of itself and then repeat.

7. With your hands, form a dough round that is about 7" in diameter and 1" thick. (If you make it any larger or flatter you will end up with hard, flat biscuits.)

8. Cut out 2" biscuits using a biscuit cutter, the mouth of a glass, or the lid of a Mason jar. Do not twist cutter when cutting; this will crimp the edges of biscuits, causing them not to rise well. Re-form dough scraps into a dough round and cut out more biscuits. Put biscuits on prepared pan or baking sheet.

9. Bake biscuits for 15–20 minutes. At the 15-minute point, check to see if biscuits are golden brown. In a small bowl, melt remaining 2 tablespoons buttery spread and brush on top of warm biscuits. Serve warm. Store leftovers in an airtight container for up to 3 days.

Lemon Blueberry Scones

Ingredients :

SCONES
- ½ cup dairy-free buttery spread
- 1 tablespoon white vinegar
- ¾ cup plus 2 tablespoons unsweetened almond milk, divided
- 3 cups plus 2 tablespoons gluten-free all-purpose flour with xanthan gum
- ⅓ cup sugar
- 2 tablespoons gluten-free baking powder

- ½ teaspoon salt
- 1 tablespoon dried lemon peel
- 2 large eggs, whisked
- 1 cup frozen blueberries

LEMON GLAZE
- 1 cup confectioners' sugar
- 1 tablespoon lemon juice
- ½ teaspoon pure vanilla extract
- 1 tablespoon water

Directions :

1. Preheat oven to 425°F. Line a baking sheet with parchment paper.
2. Cut buttery spread into small pieces and freeze for 10 minutes. Combine vinegar and cup milk in a small bowl and set aside 2–5 minutes in the refrigerator.
3. In a large bowl, add flour, sugar, baking powder, salt, and lemon peel and stir to combine.
4. Cut buttery spread into flour mixture with a pastry cutter or fork until it looks like small peas. Add milk mixture and eggs and stir until a soft, sticky dough forms. Carefully stir in blueberries.
5. Add 1 tablespoon flour to a piece of parchment paper. Place dough on top of the floured parchment paper. Dust the top of dough with remaining 1 tablespoon flour and fold dough over on itself two times.
6. With your hands, form a dough round that is about 7" in diameter and 2" thick. If you make it any larger or flatter you will end up with flat scones.
7. Run a sharp knife under warm water and cut dough round in half. Then cut each half into four slices. You will now have eight dough triangles. Carefully place dough on prepared baking sheet. Brush the tops of dough with remaining 2 tablespoons milk. Bake for 15–20 minutes until the tops are golden brown.
8. Add the glaze ingredients to a small bowl and stir together until smooth. Drizzle over warm scones. Store in an airtight container for up to 3 days.

Jam-Filled Danish

Ingredients :
- ¼ cup warm water (110°F to 115°F) plus 5 tablespoons water, divided
- ½ cup plus 1 tablespoon granulated sugar, divided
- 1 packet (2¼ teaspoons) instant yeast
- 2 cups plus 2 tablespoons gluten-free all-purpose flour with xanthan gum, divided
- 1 teaspoon salt
- ½ cup dairy-free buttery spread

- 2 large eggs, yolks and whites divided
- ½ cup unsweetened almond milk
- ¼ teaspoon plus ⅛ teaspoon pure vanilla extract, divided
- ¼ teaspoon plus ⅛ teaspoon pure almond extract, divided
- 8 teaspoons gluten-free raspberry jam
- 1 cup confectioners' sugar

Directions :

1. Add ¼ cup warm water and 1 tablespoon granulated sugar to a small bowl. Pour in the yeast and allow to sit for 2–3 minutes until foamy.

2. In a large bowl, add 2 cups flour, ½ cup sugar, and salt. Cut in buttery spread with a pastry cutter or fork until it looks like small peas.

3. Separate eggs and place whites in a small bowl, cover, and place in the refrigerator.

4. Add yeast mixture, yolks, milk, ¼ teaspoon vanilla, and ¼ teaspoon almond extract to flour mixture and mix until smooth. Cover the bowl and place in the freezer for 30 minutes.

5. Add 1 tablespoon flour to a large piece of parchment paper. Place dough on the floured parchment paper. Dust the top of dough with 1 tablespoon flour and fold dough in half on top of itself and then in half on itself again.

6. Form the dough into a round 7" in diameter and 1" thick. Cut out dough using a greased 3" biscuit cutter. Do not twist cutter when cutting; this will crimp the edges of the dough, causing it not to rise well. Put dough rounds on a baking sheet lined with parchment paper, cover with a kitchen towel, and let rise in a warm place for 30 minutes.

7. Use the back of a rounded tablespoon to press down on the center of each dough round. Place 1 teaspoon of jam in the center of each. Add 1 tablespoon water to the egg whites and whisk. Brush the tops of dough with the egg white mixture.

8. Bake for 18–20 minutes until the tops start to turn golden brown. In a small bowl, whisk together confectioners' sugar, 1/8 teaspoon vanilla extract, 1/8 teaspoon pure almond extract, and remaining 4 tablespoons water. Drizzle glaze on top. Allow Danish to cool for 5–10 minutes until jam is no longer hot before serving.

Cinnamon Biscuits

Ingredients :

BISCUITS
- 6 tablespoons dairy-free buttery spread
- 1 tablespoon white vinegar
- 1 cup unsweetened almond milk
- 2 cups plus 2 tablespoons gluten-free all-purpose flour with xanthan gum

- 1 tablespoon gluten-free baking powder
- 1 teaspoon salt
- 2 tablespoons granulated sugar
- 1 large egg, whisked
- ¼ cup light brown sugar, packed
- 1 tablespoon ground cinnamon

GLAZE
- 1 cup confectioners' sugar
- 1 teaspoon pure vanilla extract
- 2 teaspoons unsweetened almond milk

Directions :

1. Preheat oven to 450°F.
2. Cut buttery spread into small pieces and put in the freezer for 10 minutes. In a small bowl, add vinegar and milk and let stand 2–5 minutes in the refrigerator to keep cold.
3. In a large bowl, add 2 cups flour, baking powder, salt, and sugar and stir. Cut in buttery spread into the flour mixture with a pastry cutter or fork until it looks like small peas.
4. Add in the milk mixture and egg and stir until a soft dough forms. Do not overmix. The dough will be sticky. Do not roll out dough.
5. Add 1 tablespoon flour to a large piece of parchment paper. Place dough on top of floured parchment paper. Form a dough round that is 7" in diameter and 1" thick.
6. In a small bowl, add brown sugar and cinnamon and stir to combine. Sprinkle 2 tablespoons sugar mixture all over the top of dough round.
7. Gently fold dough over on itself. Sprinkle another 2 tablespoons sugar mixture over dough. Fold dough in half on top of itself again.
8. With your hands form a dough round 7" in diameter and 1" thick. Sprinkle remaining sugar mixture over dough round.
9. Grease a large cast-iron pan with vegetable oil or line a baking sheet with parchment paper. Cut out twelve 2" biscuits using a biscuit cutter or the mouth of a glass. Do not twist cutter when cutting. Put biscuits on prepared pan or baking sheet.
10. Bake biscuits for 15–20 minutes. At the 15-minute point, check to see if they are golden brown.
11. In a small bowl, stir glaze ingredients until smooth. Spread over biscuits and serve warm. Store in an airtight container for up to 3 days.

Homemade Bagels

Ingredients :

- 2¼ cups plus 1 tablespoon water, warmed to 100°F–110°F
- 1 tablespoon instant yeast
- 1 tablespoon granulated sugar
- 3½ cups gluten-free all-purpose flour with xanthan gum
- 3 tablespoons psyllium husk powder
- 2 teaspoons gluten-free baking powder
- 1½ teaspoons salt
- 1 tablespoon light brown sugar, packed
- 1 cup dairy-free buttery spread, melted
- 1 teaspoon apple cider vinegar
- ¼ cup honey
- 1 large egg white, whisked

Directions :

1. Preheat oven to 200°F. Once it gets to 100°F, turn off the oven.

2. Combine water, yeast, and granulated sugar in the bowl of a stand-up mixer fitted with a dough hook. Stir; let stand 5 minutes until foamy.

3. Add flour, psyllium husk powder, baking powder, salt, and brown sugar and mix until fully combined. Add buttery spread and vinegar and beat on low speed for 2 minutes. Raise the mixer speed to medium and knead for 5 minutes.

4. Place dough in an ovenproof bowl sprayed with gluten-free nonstick cooking spray. Cover the bowl with plastic wrap and then a kitchen towel. Allow dough to rise for 20 minutes in the warm oven.

5. Line a baking sheet with parchment paper. Turn dough out onto parchment paper and cut into eight pieces. Roll each piece into a ball. Press your finger through the center of each ball to make a hole about 1" in diameter. Cover the shaped bagels with a kitchen towel and let rise on the counter for 10 minutes.

6. Preheat oven to 425°F.

7. Fill a large pot with 2 quarts water. Whisk in honey. Bring water to a boil, then reduce heat to medium-high. Drop bagels in one at a time. Cook bagels for 30 seconds on each side. Remove with a slotted spoon and return boiled bagels to the sheet, right side up, with flat bottoms against pan.

8. Whisk the egg white and 1 tablespoon water together in a small bowl. Brush the tops of bagels with egg wash on top and around the sides. Bake for 7 minutes and then rotate the pan and cook for another 8 minutes until golden brown and internal temperature reaches 180°F. Remove from the oven and allow bagels to cool on the baking sheet for 10 minutes before serving. Store in an airtight container for up to 3 days.

Rosemary Focaccia Bread

Ingredients :

- 2½ cups plus 1 tablespoon gluten-free all-purpose flour with xanthan gum
- 1 packet (2¼ teaspoons) instant yeast
- 1 tablespoon gluten-free baking powder
- 2 teaspoons salt, divided
- 1½ teaspoons dried rosemary, divided
- 1 tablespoon honey
- 1½ cups warm water (110°F–115°F)
- 1 teaspoon apple cider vinegar
- 1 cup olive oil, divided

Directions :

1. Preheat oven to 200°F. Once it gets to 100°F, turn off oven.
2. In a large bowl, combine flour, yeast, baking powder, ½ teaspoon salt, and 1 teaspoon rosemary. Stir to combine ingredients.
3. Add honey to warm water and stir until honey is dissolved.
4. Pour the warm water mixture into the flour mixture and mix with your mixer with a dough hook or paddle attachment on low.
5. Pour vinegar and ½ cup olive oil into the dough mixture and mix on medium speed for 3 minutes. The dough will be very sticky.
6. Place dough in an ovenproof bowl sprayed with gluten-free nonstick cooking spray. Cover the bowl with plastic wrap and then with a kitchen towel and place in warm oven for 30 minutes to rise.
7. Remove dough from the oven and preheat oven to 425°F. Coat a jelly pan with ¼ cup olive oil. Put dough onto the pan and begin pressing it out to fit the size of the pan. Using your fingers make impressions throughout the dough, but do not poke holes. Spread the remaining ¼ cup olive on top of the dough. Sprinkle with remaining 1 teaspoon salt and ½ teaspoon rosemary. Bake for 20 minutes until golden brown. Allow to cool for 3–5 minutes before slicing the bread. Store in an airtight container for up to 3 days.

Soft Pretzels

Ingredients :
- ½ cup unsweetened almond milk, warm (100°F–110°F)
- 1 teaspoon granulated sugar
- 1 packet (2¼ teaspoons) instant yeast
- 3⅓ cups plus 1 tablespoon gluten-free all-purpose flour with xanthan gum, divided
- 1½ teaspoons gluten-free baking powder
- 1½ teaspoons salt
- 1 cup dairy-free plain coconut yogurt
- 2 large eggs, divided

- 6 tablespoons baking soda
- 1 tablespoon coarse sea salt

Directions :

1. Preheat oven to 200°F. Once it gets to 100°F turn off oven.

2. In a small bowl, stir together milk, sugar, and yeast. Let stand for 5–10 minutes until foamy. In a large bowl, combine flour, baking powder, and salt. In a separate small bowl, whisk together yogurt and one egg.

3. Add the yeast mixture and yogurt mixture to the flour mixture. Mix together until it forms a sticky dough.

4. Add dough to an ovenproof bowl sprayed with gluten-free nonstick cooking spray. Cover the bowl with plastic wrap and a kitchen towel, and place in the warm oven for 30 minutes.

5. Add 1 tablespoon flour to a piece of parchment paper. Turn out dough onto the parchment paper and divide into eight balls.

6. Take each piece of dough and begin rolling them into a long rope, about the length of the parchment paper (11"). Take the ends of the dough rope and bring them together so the dough forms a circle. Twist the ends over each other twice, then bring them toward yourself and press them down into a pretzel shape.

7. Preheat oven to 450°F and line a baking sheet with parchment paper. Add 2 quarts water in a large pot and stir in baking soda. Bring water to a boil, then reduce heat to medium-high. Drop pretzels in the boiling water one at a time and boil for 30 seconds. Using a wire skimmer or slotted spoon, return pretzels to the sheet, right side up, with flat bottoms against the sheet. Repeat until all pretzels have been boiled.

8. In a small bowl, whisk remaining egg. Brush pretzels with egg and sprinkle with salt. Bake for 15 minutes or until golden brown. Allow to cool for 2–3 minutes and serve warm.

Flatbread

Ingredients :
- 1 packet (2¼ teaspoons) instant yeast
- 1 tablespoon honey
- 1½ cups warm water (100°F–110°F)
- 1 tablespoon gluten-free baking powder
- 1 teaspoon salt
- 1 teaspoon apple cider vinegar
- ¼ cup plus 2 tablespoons olive oil, divided
- 3 cups plus 1 tablespoon gluten-free all-purpose flour with xanthan gum, divided

Directions :

1. Preheat oven to 200°F. Once it gets to 100°F, turn off oven.

2. In the bowl of a stand-up mixer fitted with a dough hook, combine the yeast, honey, and water; mix until combined. Let yeast sit for 5 minutes until foamy.

3. Add baking powder, salt, vinegar, and ¼ cup olive oil and mix. Add 3 cups flour, 1 cup at a time, mixing at the lowest speed until all the flour has been incorporated and dough pulls away from the side of the bowl, about 4 minutes.

4. Place dough in a greased ovenproof bowl covered with plastic wrap and then a kitchen towel and let rise in a warm oven for 30 minutes.

5. Flour a piece of parchment paper with remaining 1 tablespoon flour. Divide dough into eight pieces and flatten them out with the palms of your hands, then use a rolling pin to roll each piece into a thin circle.

6. Heat remaining 2 tablespoons olive oil in a large skillet over medium-high heat. Once the skillet is hot, place dough into the skillet. Cook for 1 minute. When the edges are starting to look golden, flip the bread carefully with a spatula and cook for another minute. Remove to a plate and cover with aluminum foil to keep warm. Store in an airtight container for up to 3 days.

Homemade Popovers

Ingredients :
- 2 large eggs
- 1 cup gluten-free all-purpose flour with xanthan gum
- ½ teaspoon salt
- 1 cup unsweetened almond milk

Directions :

1. Preheat oven to 450°F and grease a twelve-cup popover pan with gluten-free nonstick cooking spray.

2. In a large bowl, beat eggs. Beat in flour, salt, and milk until smooth.

3. Fill baking cups three-quarters full and bake for 20 minutes. Decrease the oven temperature to 350°F and bake for 20 minutes longer until golden brown. Do not open the oven during the baking process. Remove popovers immediately from the baking cups and serve immediately while hot. Store in an airtight container for up to 3 days.

Herbed Crusty Bread

Ingredients :
- 3 cups gluten-free all-purpose flour with xanthan gum, divided
- 1 tablespoon granulated sugar
- 1 teaspoon salt
- 1 packet (2¼ teaspoons) instant yeast
- 1½ cups warm water (110°F)

- ¼ cup dairy-free buttery spread
- 2 large eggs, room temperature and beaten
- 1 teaspoon apple cider vinegar
- ½ teaspoon dried rosemary
- ¼ teaspoon dried thyme
- ¼ teaspoon garlic powder

Directions :

1. Preheat oven to 200°F. Once it gets to 100°F, turn off your oven.

2. In a large bowl, combine 2 cups flour, sugar, salt, and yeast. Add water, buttery spread, eggs, vinegar, rosemary, thyme, and garlic powder and beat on low 1 minute. Stir in remaining 1 cup flour; beat 2 minutes on medium.

3. Transfer dough to a greased 9" × 5" pan. Cover with plastic wrap and then a kitchen towel and place in the warm oven for 30 minutes to rise. Remove from the oven and keep covered. Preheat oven to 375°F. Bake for 40–45 minutes. Remove from pan and cool on a wire rack for 20 minutes before slicing and serving warm.

Lemon Blueberry Quick Bread

- **Ingredients :**
- ⅓ cup dairy-free buttery spread, melted
- 2 large eggs, whisked
- 1 teaspoon pure vanilla extract
- 1 tablespoon gluten-free lemon extract
- 1½ cups gluten-free all-purpose flour with xanthan gum
- ½ cup sugar
- 1 teaspoon baking soda
- ½ teaspoon gluten-free baking powder
- ¼ teaspoon salt
- 1 cup unsweetened almond milk
- 1 cup frozen blueberries

Directions :

1. Preheat oven to 350°F. Spray a 4" × 8" loaf pan with gluten-free nonstick cooking spray.

2. In a large bowl, add buttery spread, eggs, vanilla extract, and lemon extract and stir to combine ingredients. Add flour, sugar, baking soda, baking powder, and salt to the mixture and mix until fully combined. Add milk and mix until smooth. Fold in blueberries. Pour batter into prepared loaf pan.

3. Bake on the center rack for 50 minutes to 1 hour or until a toothpick inserted in the center comes out clean. Allow the bread to cool for 3–5 minutes before removing from the pan and slicing. Store leftovers in an airtight container at room temperature for up to 3 days.

Garlic Breadsticks

Ingredients :
- 2½ cups plus 1 tablespoon gluten-free all-purpose flour with xanthan gum
- 1 packet (2¼ teaspoons) instant yeast
- 1 tablespoon gluten-free baking powder
- ¼ teaspoon garlic powder
- 1 teaspoon salt
- 1 tablespoon honey
- 1½ cups warm water (110°F–115°F)
- ½ cup plus 1 teaspoon olive oil, divided
- 1 teaspoon apple cider vinegar
- 2 tablespoons dairy-free buttery spread, melted

Directions :

1. Preheat oven to 200°F. Once it gets to 100°F turn off oven.
2. In a large bowl, combine flour, yeast, baking powder, garlic powder, and salt. Stir to combine ingredients.
3. Add honey to warm water and stir until it is dissolved.
4. Pour the warm water mixture into the flour mixture and mix with your mixer with a dough hook or paddle attachment on low.
5. Pour ½ cup olive oil and vinegar into the dough mixture and mix on medium speed for 3 minutes. The dough will be very sticky.
6. Line a baking sheet with parchment paper. Pour remaining 1 teaspoon oil into a sealable plastic bag and spread around so the bag is coated. Add dough to the bag toward one of the bottom corners. Cut 1" off of the corner of the bag. Squeeze the bag toward the cut corner so the dough comes out of the corner of the bag. Pipe dough down to make a length of breadstick, about 7", on the baking sheet. Repeat piping dough into breadstick shapes until all dough is used. Place in the warm oven and let rise for 30 minutes.
7. Remove dough from the oven and preheat oven to 425°F.
8. Bake for 15 minutes until golden brown. Brush tops with melted buttery spread. Allow to cool for 1–2 minutes, then serve warm. Store in an airtight container for up to 3 days.

Marbled Quick Bread

Ingredients :
- ⅓ cup dairy-free buttery spread, melted
- 2 large eggs, whisked
- 1 tablespoon pure vanilla extract

- 1½ cups gluten-free all-purpose flour with xanthan gum
- ½ cup sugar
- 1 teaspoon baking soda
- ½ teaspoon gluten-free baking powder
- ¼ teaspoon salt
- 1 cup unsweetened almond milk
- 1 tablespoon cocoa powder

Directions :

1. Preheat oven to 350°F. Spray a 4" × 8" loaf pan with gluten-free nonstick cooking spray.
2. In a large bowl, add buttery spread, eggs, and vanilla extract, and stir to combine. Add flour, sugar, baking soda, baking powder, and salt to the mixture and mix until fully combined. Add milk and stir until smooth.
3. Add 1 cup of batter to a small bowl. Stir in cocoa powder and mix until fully combined to make chocolate batter.
4. Pour vanilla batter into prepared loaf pan. Drizzle chocolate batter on top and use a knife to swirl through the vanilla batter.
5. Bake on the center rack for 50 minutes to 1 hour or until a toothpick inserted in the center comes out clean. Allow bread to cool for 3–5 minutes before removing from the pan and slicing. Store leftovers in an airtight at room temperature container for 3 days.

Potato Rolls

Ingredients :
- ⅓ cup plus ½ cup warm water (110°F to 115°F), divided
- 1 tablespoon honey
- 1 packet (2¼ teaspoons) instant yeast
- ½ cup mashed potatoes (1 large baked potato, peeled, cooked, and mashed)
- ⅓ cup sugar
- ⅓ cup dairy-free buttery spread
- 1 large egg, room temperature
- 1¼ teaspoons salt
- 1 teaspoon apple cider vinegar
- 3 cups gluten-free all-purpose flour with xanthan gum

Directions :

1. Preheat oven to 200°F. Once it gets to 100°F, turn off oven.
2. In a large bowl, add 1/3 cup warm water, honey, and yeast. Stir to combine and allow to sit for 5 minutes until foamy.
3. Add potatoes, sugar, buttery spread, egg, salt, vinegar, flour, and remaining ½ cup water to the yeast

mixture and mix until smooth. The dough will be sticky.

4. Spray two 9" metal cake pans with gluten-free nonstick cooking spray. Using a greased ice cream scoop, make sixteen dough balls; place eight into the first pan and eight into the second pan. Cover the pans with a kitchen towel and allow to rise in the warm oven for 30 minutes. Remove from the oven and keep covered while preheating oven to 375°F.

5. Bake rolls on the middle rack for 20 minutes until light golden brown. The temperature of the rolls should measure 200°F internally. Allow rolls to cool for 1–2 minutes. Serve warm. Store in an airtight container for up to 3 days.

Cranberry Orange Quick Bread

Ingredients :
- ⅓ cup dairy-free buttery spread, melted
- 2 large eggs, whisked
- 1 teaspoon pure vanilla extract
- ¼ teaspoon pure almond extract
- ½ teaspoon dried orange peel
- 1½ cups gluten-free all-purpose flour with xanthan gum
- ½ cup sugar
- 1 teaspoon baking soda
- ½ teaspoon gluten-free baking powder
- ¼ teaspoon salt
- ½ cup unsweetened almond milk
- ½ cup orange juice
- 1 cup frozen cranberries

Directions :

1. Preheat oven to 350°F. Spray a 4" × 8" loaf pan with gluten-free nonstick cooking spray.

2. In a large bowl, add buttery spread, eggs, vanilla extract, almond extract, and orange peel and stir to combine. Add flour, sugar, baking soda, baking powder, and salt to the mixture and stir until fully combined. Add milk and orange juice and mix until smooth. Carefully fold in cranberries. Pour batter into prepared loaf pan.

3. Bake on the center rack for 50 minutes to 1 hour or until a toothpick inserted in the center comes out clean. Allow the bread to cool for 3–5 minutes before removing from the pan and slicing. Store leftovers in an airtight container at room temperature for up to 3 days.

Cream of Mushroom Soup

Ingredients :
- 2 tablespoons dairy-free buttery spread

- 1 cup finely chopped mushrooms
- ½ teaspoon jarred minced garlic
- 6 tablespoons gluten-free all-purpose flour with xanthan gum
- 1 teaspoon onion powder
- 2 cups gluten-free chicken broth
- ½ teaspoon salt
- ⅛ teaspoon ground black pepper
- ⅛ teaspoon ground nutmeg
- 1 cup unsweetened almond milk

Directions :

1. Add buttery spread, mushrooms, and garlic to a large pot and sauté over medium-high heat for 1–2 minutes until mushrooms are tender.

2. Sprinkle flour and onion powder over mushrooms and stir to coat. Stir in broth, salt, pepper, and nutmeg until flour dissolves. Bring to a boil and stir until thickened, about 2 minutes.

3. Reduce the heat to low to simmer and stir in milk. Simmer, uncovered, for about 10–15 minutes, stirring occasionally. Remove soup from the heat when it reaches desired thickness.

Savory Chicken and Rice Soup

Ingredients :
- 1 tablespoon olive oil
- 3 large carrots, peeled and diced
- 1 stalk celery, diced
- 1 teaspoon jarred minced garlic
- 1 tablespoon onion powder
- ½ teaspoon dried thyme
- 5 cups gluten-free chicken broth
- ½ teaspoon seasoned salt
- ⅛ teaspoon ground black pepper
- 2 (5-ounce) boneless, skinless chicken breasts, diced
- 1 cup long-grain white rice

Directions :

1. Heat olive oil in a large pot over medium heat. Add carrots and celery and sauté vegetables for 5–7 minutes until very tender, stirring occasionally. Add garlic, onion powder, and thyme and sauté for 30 seconds until fragrant.

2. Add broth, salt, and pepper and bring to a boil over medium-high heat. Add chicken and rice and stir to combine. Turn heat down to medium and simmer uncovered for 15–20 minutes until rice is tender. Remove from the heat and cover and let sit for 5 minutes. Serve warm.

Loaded Baked Potato Soup

Ingredients :
- 1 (12-ounce) package gluten-free bacon
- 1 cup peeled and chopped sweet onion
- 6 cups gluten-free chicken broth
- 2 pounds baking potatoes, peeled and cubed
- ⅔ cup dairy-free buttery spread
- ¾ cup gluten-free all-purpose flour with xanthan gum
- 4 cups unsweetened almond milk, divided
- 1 teaspoon salt
- ¼ teaspoon ground black pepper
- ¼ cup sliced green onion

Directions :

1. In a large skillet, cook bacon for 6–8 minutes over medium heat until crisp; set on a paper towel–lined plate. Allow to cool for 5 minutes and crumble bacon; set aside. Drain bacon grease, reserving 2 tablespoons in the skillet. Add onions and sauté over medium-high heat for 6 minutes until tender.

2. Add broth and potatoes to a large pot and bring to a boil over medium-high heat. Reduce heat to medium and simmer for 10 minutes until potatoes are fork-tender.

3. Melt buttery spread in the skillet with onions over low heat. Stir in flour and whisk until smooth. Stir in 2 cups milk and whisk until fully combined and flour is dissolved. Pour the milk mixture into the potato mixture. Add remaining 2 cups milk, salt, and pepper to the pot. Cook over medium heat for 5 minutes, stirring constantly, until the mixture has thickened.

4. Stir in the bacon and cook until thoroughly heated. Serve and garnish with green onions.

Creamy Chicken Corn Chowder

Ingredients :
- 2 tablespoons dairy-free buttery spread
- 1 teaspoon jarred minced garlic
- ⅔ cup gluten-free all-purpose flour with xanthan gum
- 1 tablespoon onion powder
- 1 teaspoon dried thyme
- 2 cups gluten-free chicken broth
- ½ teaspoon salt
- ⅛ teaspoon ground black pepper
- 2 cups peeled and diced russet potatoes
- 2 cups chopped cooked chicken

- 1 (15-ounce) can corn, drained
- 1 cup unsweetened almond milk

Directions :

1. Add buttery spread and garlic to a large pot and sauté over medium-high heat for 30 seconds until garlic is tender.

2. Sprinkle flour, onion powder, and thyme over garlic. Stir in broth, salt, and pepper. Stir the mixture until flour dissolves. Add potatoes and bring the mixture to a boil, stirring frequently, then reduce heat to medium-low and cook uncovered for 10 minutes or just until potatoes are tender. Bring soup to a boil for 2 minutes, stirring until thickened.

3. Add chicken and corn and stir to combine. Reduce the heat to low and stir in milk. Simmer uncovered for about 10–15 minutes, stirring occasionally. Remove soup from the heat when it reaches desired thickness.

Zuppa Toscana

Ingredients :
- 1 tablespoon olive oil
- 1 pound mild gluten-free Italian sausage, chopped
- ½ teaspoon crushed red pepper flakes
- 6 strips gluten-free bacon, diced
- 1 large sweet onion, peeled and chopped
- 3 tablespoons jarred minced garlic
- 4 cups gluten-free chicken broth
- 2 cups water
- 4 cups diced russet potatoes
- ½ teaspoon salt
- ¼ teaspoon ground black pepper
- 1 cup unsweetened almond milk
- 3 tablespoons gluten-free all-purpose flour with xanthan gum
- 2 cups chopped baby spinach leaves, stems removed

Directions :

1. Add olive oil, sausage, and red pepper flakes to a large pot and cook for 10–15 minutes over medium-high heat until sausage is browned. Drain excess grease and set sausage aside.

2. Add bacon, onions, and garlic to the pot and sauté for 5 minutes until bacon is browned and onions are tender.

3. Add the chicken broth, water, potatoes, salt, and pepper. Boil for 20 minutes until potatoes are fork-tender.

4. In a small bowl, whisk together milk and flour. Reduce the heat to medium and stir in the milk

mixture and cooked sausage and cook for 5 minutes. Stir spinach into soup just before serving.

Cream of Chicken Soup

Ingredients :
- 2 tablespoons dairy-free buttery spread
- ½ teaspoon jarred minced garlic
- 6 tablespoons gluten-free all-purpose flour with xanthan gum
- 1 teaspoon onion powder
- 1 teaspoon dried thyme
- 2 cups gluten-free chicken broth
- ½ teaspoon salt
- ⅛ teaspoon ground black pepper
- ⅛ teaspoon ground nutmeg
- 2 cups chopped cooked chicken
- 1 cup unsweetened almond milk

Directions :

1. Add buttery spread and garlic to a large pot and sauté over medium-high heat for 30 seconds until garlic is tender.

2. Sprinkle in flour, onion powder, and thyme. Stir in broth, salt, pepper, and nutmeg until flour dissolves. Bring to a boil and stir until thickened, about 2 minutes.

3. Add chicken to soup and stir to combine. Reduce the heat to low to simmer and stir in milk. Simmer uncovered for about 10–15 minutes, stirring occasionally.

Hearty Hamburger Soup

Ingredients :
- 1 teaspoon olive oil
- 1 pound 90/10 ground beef
- 1 medium sweet onion, peeled and chopped
- 1 cup chopped celery
- 1½ teaspoons jarred minced garlic
- 6 cups gluten-free beef broth
- 1 (14-ounce) can diced tomatoes, including liquid
- 1 (8-ounce) can tomato sauce
- 1 teaspoon Italian seasoning
- 1½ teaspoons salt
- ¼ teaspoon ground black pepper
- 2 medium russet potatoes, peeled and cubed
- 3 cups frozen mixed vegetables

Directions :

1. Add olive oil, beef, onions, celery, and garlic to a large pot and cook over medium-high heat for 5–7 minutes until meat is browned. Drain excess fat.
2. Add broth, tomatoes, tomato sauce, Italian seasoning, salt, pepper, potatoes, and mixed vegetables. Stir to combine, then bring to a boil. Reduce the heat, cover the pot, and simmer for 20–25 minutes until potatoes are fork-tender.

Italian Vegetable Soup

Ingredients :
- 1 tablespoon olive oil
- 2 (14-ounce) cans petite-diced tomatoes, including liquid
- 1 tablespoon garlic powder
- 1 tablespoon onion powder
- 1 tablespoon dried basil
- 1 teaspoon salt
- 2 gluten-free beef bouillon cubes
- 1 (16-ounce) can kidney beans
- 1 (16-ounce) can cannellini beans
- 1 (16-ounce) can great northern beans
- 1 cup peeled and chopped carrots
- 1 cup chopped trimmed green beans
- 1 large zucchini, diced
- 1 large yellow squash, diced
- 1 (10-ounce) package baby spinach
- 1 cup water

Directions :

1. Add olive oil into the bottom of a slow cooker. Add remaining ingredients and stir. Cook on high for hours until vegetables are softened.

Southern Ham and Bean Soup

Ingredients :
- 1 tablespoon olive oil
- 1 small sweet onion, peeled and finely chopped
- 1 teaspoon jarred minced garlic
- 2 cups diced cooked ham
- 2 teaspoons dried thyme
- 2 (15-ounce) cans white beans, drained and rinsed

- 4 cups gluten-free chicken broth
- 1 teaspoon seasoned salt
- ⅛ teaspoon ground black pepper

Directions :

1. Add olive oil, onions, garlic, ham, and thyme to a large pot over medium-high heat and cook for 4 minutes until onions are softened, stirring occasionally.

2. Add beans, broth, salt, and pepper and simmer uncovered for 20 minutes, stirring occasionally. Serve warm.

Chicken Fajita Soup

Ingredients :

- 1 teaspoon olive oil
- 1 large green bell pepper, seeded and chopped
- 1 large red bell pepper, seeded and chopped
- 1 cup peeled and chopped sweet onion
- 1 tablespoon jarred minced garlic
- 1 pound boneless, skinless chicken breasts
- 1 (15-ounce) can black beans, rinsed and drained
- 1 (15-ounce) can fire-roasted diced tomatoes, drained
- 5 cups gluten-free chicken broth
- 1 teaspoon chili powder
- 1 teaspoon paprika
- 1 teaspoon ground cumin
- ½ teaspoon dried oregano
- 1 teaspoon salt
- ¼ teaspoon ground black pepper
- 1 cup dry long-grain white rice
- 2 cups water
- ¼ cup chopped fresh cilantro

Directions :

1. Add olive oil, bell peppers, onions, and garlic in a large pot and sauté over medium-high heat for 3–5 minutes until vegetables are softened.

2. Add chicken, black beans, tomatoes, broth, seasonings, rice, and water and stir to combine. Bring to a boil, then lower the heat and simmer for 20 minutes.

3. Use tongs to remove cooked chicken breasts to a plate, cool for 5 minutes, then shred with two forks. Continue simmering for 10–15 minutes until rice is tender. Add shredded chicken back to soup and stir to combine. Serve garnished with cilantro.

French Onion Soup

Ingredients :
- ½ cup dairy-free buttery spread
- 4 large sweet onions, peeled and thinly sliced
- 1 teaspoon jarred minced garlic
- 2 bay leaves
- 2 teaspoons dried thyme
- ½ teaspoon salt
- ¼ teaspoon ground black pepper
- 1 cup dry white wine
- 3 tablespoons gluten-free all-purpose flour with xanthan gum
- 8 cups gluten-free beef broth

Directions :

1. Melt buttery spread in a large pot over medium heat. Add onions, garlic, bay leaves, thyme, salt, and pepper and cook for 20–25 minutes until onions are very soft and caramelized.

2. Add wine and bring to a boil, then reduce heat to medium and simmer 5 minutes. Remove bay leaves. Sprinkle mixture with flour and stir. Reduce heat to medium-low and cook 10 minutes.

3. Add beef broth and bring soup back to a simmer. Cook for 10 minutes.

Classic Tomato Soup

Ingredients :
- 4 tablespoons dairy-free buttery spread
- ½ large sweet onion, peeled and sliced
- 1½ cups gluten-free chicken stock
- 1 (28-ounce) can peeled tomatoes, including liquid
- ½ teaspoon salt
- 1 teaspoon granulated sugar

Directions :

1. Melt buttery spread in a large pot over medium heat. Add onions, stock, tomatoes, salt, and sugar and stir to combine. Bring to a simmer and cook uncovered for 40 minutes, stirring occasionally.

2. Blend with an immersion blender or transfer to a blender and blend in batches until smooth and well combined. Serve warm.

Butternut Squash Soup

Ingredients :
- 2 tablespoons dairy-free buttery spread

- 1 medium sweet onion, peeled and chopped
- 1 (3-pound) butternut squash, peeled, seeded, and diced
- 4 cups gluten-free chicken stock
- 1 tablespoon pure maple syrup
- ⅛ teaspoon ground nutmeg
- ½ teaspoon salt
- ¼ teaspoon ground black pepper

Directions :

1. In a large pot, melt the buttery spread over medium heat. Add onions and cook for 6–8 minutes until translucent. Add squash and stock. Bring to a simmer and cook for 15–20 minutes until squash is tender.
2. Remove squash with a slotted spoon and place in a blender and purée. Return blended squash to the pot. Stir in maple syrup, nutmeg, salt, and pepper. Serve.

Ramen Soup with Eggs

Ingredients :

- 2 teaspoons sesame oil
- 1 tablespoon jarred minced ginger
- 1 tablespoon jarred minced garlic
- ½ cup sliced shitake mushrooms
- 3 tablespoons gluten-free soy sauce
- 1 tablespoon rice wine vinegar
- 6 cups gluten-free chicken stock
- 4 servings gluten-free ramen noodles (4 cubes dried ramen)
- 2 large soft-boiled eggs, halved
- ¼ cup sliced green onion

Directions :

1. Heat oil in a large pot over medium heat. Add ginger and garlic and sauté for 30 seconds until fragrant. Add mushrooms and sauté for 2 minutes until tender. Add soy sauce and vinegar and stir to combine. Add stock, cover, and bring to a boil. Remove the lid and let simmer uncovered for 2 minutes.
2. Add ramen noodles to pot and cook according to the package directions until soft. Divide noodles into four bowls, pour in broth, and top with a half of a soft-boiled egg and green onions.

Taco Soup

Ingredients :

- 1 teaspoon olive oil
- 1 tablespoon jarred minced garlic
- 1 pound 90/10 ground beef
- 1 tablespoon onion powder
- 2 teaspoons chili powder
- ½ teaspoon dried oregano
- 1 teaspoon ground cumin
- ½ teaspoon paprika
- 1 teaspoon salt
- ⅛ teaspoon ground black pepper
- 1 (28-ounce) can crushed tomatoes, including liquid
- 1 (4-ounce) can diced green chiles
- 1 (15-ounce) can kidney beans, drained and rinsed
- 1 (15-ounce) can black beans, drained and rinsed
- 1 (15-ounce) can corn, drained
- 2 cups gluten-free beef broth
- 1 cup crushed gluten-free corn chips

Directions :

1. In a large pot, heat olive oil over medium heat. Add garlic and sauté for 30 seconds until tender. Add beef and cook for 5–7 minutes, stirring frequently, until beef is brown and crumbled; drain excess fat. Add remaining ingredients except corn chips and stir to combine. Bring to a boil, then reduce heat and simmer for 20 minutes.

2. Garnish with crushed corn chips to serve.

Maryland-Style Cream of Crab Soup

- **Ingredients :**
- ½ cup dairy-free buttery spread
- ½ cup peeled and minced sweet onion
- ½ cup gluten-free all-purpose flour with xanthan gum
- 1 tablespoon Old Bay Seasoning
- 4 cups unsweetened almond milk
- 1 pound lump crabmeat, drained and picked over to remove any shells
- 3 tablespoons cooking sherry

Directions :

1. Melt buttery spread in a medium saucepan over medium heat. Add onions; cook and stir 5 minutes until softened. Add flour and Old Bay Seasoning and whisk until well blended. Pour in milk and whisk constantly, bringing to a boil.

2. Stir in crabmeat. Reduce heat to low; simmer for 20 minutes, stirring occasionally. Stir in sherry and

cook for 1 minute. Serve.

White Chicken Chili

Ingredients :
- 1 tablespoon olive oil
- 2 (6-ounce) boneless, skinless chicken breasts, cut into 1" pieces
- 1 large sweet onion, peeled and chopped
- 1 teaspoon jarred minced garlic
- 5 cups gluten-free chicken broth
- 3 (15-ounce) cans cannellini (white kidney) beans, rinsed and drained
- 2 (4-ounce) cans chopped green chiles
- 1 tablespoon dried oregano
- 2 teaspoons ground cumin
- ½ teaspoon salt
- ¼ cup chopped fresh cilantro

Directions :

1. Heat olive oil in a large pot over medium heat. Add chicken, onions, and garlic. Cook for 5–8 minutes until chicken is browned.

2. Add the broth, beans, chiles, oregano, cumin, and salt. Bring the mixture to a simmer and cook for 20–30 minutes until chicken is no longer pink and is cooked through. Divide into four bowls and top with cilantro.

New England Clam Chowder

Ingredients :
- 6 strips thick-cut gluten-free bacon, diced
- 2 tablespoons dairy-free buttery spread
- 2 celery stalks, chopped
- 1 medium sweet onion, peeled and finely diced
- 1 teaspoon jarred minced garlic
- 2 cups gluten-free chicken broth
- 3 cups peeled and diced russet potatoes
- 1 (8-ounce) bottle clam juice
- 2 bay leaves
- ½ teaspoon dried parsley
- ¼ teaspoon dried thyme
- ½ cup gluten-free all-purpose flour with xanthan gum
- 1 cup unsweetened almond milk
- 2 (10-ounce) cans chopped clams in juice

Directions :

1. In a large pot, cook bacon for 3–5 minutes over medium heat until crisp. Remove to paper towels to drain; set aside. Add buttery spread and sauté celery and onions for 3–5 minutes until tender. Add garlic; sauté for 1 minute.

2. Add broth, potatoes, clam juice, bay leaves, parsley, and thyme. Bring to a boil. Reduce heat to medium and simmer uncovered for 15–20 minutes until potatoes are fork-tender.

3. In a small bowl, whisk together flour and milk until smooth, and gradually stir the mixture into soup. Bring to a boil, stirring frequently, and cook for 1–2 minutes until thickened. Stir in clams and remove bay leaves. Crumble cooked bacon and sprinkle over each serving.

Mexican Pork Posole

Ingredients :
- 2 tablespoons olive oil
- 1 large sweet onion, peeled and chopped
- 1 jalapeño, seeded and chopped (about 1 tablespoon)
- 2 teaspoons jarred minced garlic
- 4 cups gluten-free chicken broth, divided
- 2 (4-ounce) cans green chiles, drained
- ½ cup chopped fresh cilantro leaves
- 2 teaspoons ground cumin, divided
- ½ teaspoon dried oregano
- ½ teaspoon paprika
- 1 (15-ounce) can white hominy, rinsed and drained
- 1 (15-ounce) can pinto beans, rinsed and drained
- 2 cups shredded cooked pork
- 1 tablespoon lime juice

Directions :

1. Heat olive oil in a large skillet over medium heat. Add onions and jalapeño and cook for 5 minutes or until onions are tender, stirring occasionally. Stir in garlic and cook for 30 seconds until fragrant. Spoon the onion mixture into a blender. Add ½ cup broth, chiles, and cilantro to the blender. Cover and blend until the mixture is smooth.

2. Cook the blended onion mixture and 1 teaspoon cumin in a large saucepan over medium heat for 5 minutes or until thickened, stirring often. Stir in the remaining broth, remaining cumin, oregano, paprika, hominy, and beans and heat to a boil. Reduce the heat to medium-low. Add pork and cook for 5 minutes, stirring occasionally. Stir in lime juice. Serve warm.

Stuffed Pepper Soup

- **Ingredients :**
- 1 teaspoon olive oil
- 1 pound 90/10 ground beef
- ½ teaspoon salt
- ⅛ teaspoon ground black pepper
- 1 large green bell pepper, seeded and diced
- 1 large red bell pepper, seeded and diced
- 1 cup peeled and diced sweet onion
- 2 teaspoons jarred minced garlic
- 1 (28-ounce) can diced tomatoes, undrained
- 1 (15-ounce) can tomato sauce
- 2 cups gluten-free beef broth
- 1 tablespoon light brown sugar, packed
- 1 teaspoon dried basil
- 1 teaspoon dried oregano
- 2 cups cooked long grain white rice

Directions :

1. In a large pot, heat olive oil over medium heat. Add beef, salt, and black pepper. Cook for 7–8 minutes, stirring occasionally while breaking up beef, until browned. Drain beef of excess fat and add bell peppers, onions, and garlic. Cook for 2–3 minutes until onion is translucent.

2. Add tomatoes, tomato sauce, broth, brown sugar, basil, and oregano and stir to combine. Cover and simmer for 30 minutes until peppers are tender. Add cooked rice to soup, stir to combine, and cook for 10 minutes uncovered. Serve.

Maple Bacon Sweet Potato Soup

- **Ingredients :**
- 2 tablespoons dairy-free buttery spread
- 1 cup peeled and diced sweet onion
- 8 cups peeled and chopped sweet potato
- 2 cups gluten-free chicken broth
- 2 teaspoons ground cinnamon
- ½ teaspoon ground nutmeg
- ½ teaspoon salt
- ⅛ teaspoon ground black pepper
- 4 tablespoons pure maple syrup
- 6 strips cooked gluten-free bacon, crumbled

Directions :

1. In a large pot, melt buttery spread over medium heat. Add in onions and sauté for 1–2 minutes until tender. Add in sweet potatoes, broth, and spices. Cover and bring to a boil. Let simmer for 15–20

minutes until potatoes have softened. Add maple syrup and stir.

2. Blend with an immersion blender or transfer to a blender and blend in batches until smooth and well combined. Serve topped with crumbled bacon.

Black Bean Soup

Ingredients :
- 1 teaspoon olive oil
- 6 strips gluten-free bacon, finely chopped
- 1 medium sweet onion, peeled and chopped
- 2 tablespoons jarred minced garlic
- 1 cup gluten-free chicken broth
- 1½ cups canned chopped tomatoes, including liquid
- 2 tablespoons ketchup
- 2 teaspoons gluten-free Worcestershire sauce
- ¼ teaspoon salt
- ⅛ teaspoon ground black pepper
- 1 tablespoon chili powder
- 4 (15.5-ounce) cans black beans, drained and rinsed
- 2 tablespoons lime juice
- ½ cup chopped cilantro

Directions :

1. Add olive oil in a large pot over medium heat. Add bacon and cook for 3–4 minutes. Stir in onions and cook for 3–4 minutes, stirring occasionally, until translucent. Stir in garlic and cook for 1 minute until fragrant.

2. Add broth, tomatoes, ketchup, Worcestershire sauce, salt, pepper, and chili powder. Stir in beans, turn the heat to high and bring to a low boil. Add lime juice and cook for 10 minutes. Serve with chopped cilantro.

Chicken Pot Pie Soup

Ingredients :
- 2 tablespoons dairy-free buttery spread
- 1 cup peeled and diced russet potatoes
- 1 cup peeled and chopped sweet onion
- ½ cup chopped celery
- 1 cup peeled and chopped carrots
- ½ cup gluten-free all-purpose flour with xanthan gum
- ½ teaspoon salt
- ¼ teaspoon ground black pepper

- 2 cups gluten-free chicken broth
- 1 cup frozen corn
- 1 cup frozen peas
- 2 cups shredded cooked chicken

Directions :

1. Heat buttery spread in a large pot over medium-high heat. Add potatoes, onions, celery, and carrots; cook and stir for 5–7 minutes until onions are tender.

2. Stir in flour, salt, and pepper until combined; whisk in broth. Bring to a boil over high heat, stirring occasionally.

3. Reduce heat; simmer uncovered for 10–15 minutes or until potatoes are fork-tender. Stir in corn, peas, and chicken and cook for 5–10 minutes until vegetables are heated through.

Egg Drop Soup

Ingredients :

- 3 cups gluten-free chicken broth
- 1 teaspoon ground ginger
- ¼ teaspoon garlic powder
- ½ teaspoon gluten-free soy sauce
- ½ teaspoon toasted sesame oil
- 1 tablespoon cornstarch
- 2 tablespoons cold water
- 3 large eggs, whisked
- 1 green onion, sliced

Directions :

1. In a large saucepan, add broth, ginger, garlic powder, soy sauce, and sesame oil and bring to a boil over medium heat.

2. In a small bowl, whisk together cornstarch and water until cornstarch is dissolved. Slowly pour the mixture into broth and stir. Bring to a boil; cook and stir for 2 minutes or until thickened.

3. Reduce heat and simmer for 1–2 minutes. Slowly pour whisked eggs into hot broth, stirring constantly. The egg will spread and feather. Remove from the heat; stir in onions and serve immediately.

Tex-Mex Chicken Noodle Soup

Ingredients :

- 1 tablespoon olive oil
- 1 large sweet onion, peeled and diced
- 2 teaspoons jarred minced garlic
- 1 medium carrot, peeled and sliced into half-moons
- 1 (15-ounce) can corn, drained
- 1 tablespoon dried oregano
- 1 tablespoon ground cumin
- 2 teaspoons chili powder
- ½ teaspoon salt
- 1 (15-ounce) can diced tomatoes, including liquid
- 6 cups gluten-free chicken broth
- 1 (12-ounce) box gluten-free rotini pasta
- 2 cups shredded cooked chicken
- 2 tablespoons lime juice
- ¼ cup chopped fresh cilantro

Directions :

1. Heat olive oil in a large pot over medium heat. Add onions and cook for 2 minutes until soft. Add garlic, carrots, and corn and stir until combined. Add oregano, cumin, chili powder, and salt and stir to combine.

2. Add tomatoes and chicken broth and simmer. Add pasta and cook to al dente according to the package directions. Add chicken and lime juice and stir to combine. Cook for 2 minutes. Serve topped with cilantro.

Crispy Baked Buffalo Wings

Ingredients :
- 4 pounds chicken wings, wingettes, and drumettes
- ½ cup gluten-free baking powder
- 1 teaspoon garlic powder
- ½ teaspoon salt
- ⅛ teaspoon ground black pepper
- ½ cup Frank's RedHot Sauce
- 4 tablespoons dairy-free buttery spread
- 1 tablespoon honey
- 1½ teaspoons cornstarch
- 1 tablespoon water

Directions :

1. Adjust oven rack to the middle position. Preheat oven to 450°F. Line a rimmed baking sheet with

aluminum foil, set a heatproof wire rack on the pan, and spray the rack with gluten-free nonstick cooking spray.

2. Pat wings dry with paper towels. Place wings in a large sealable plastic bag. Add baking powder, garlic powder, salt, and pepper and seal the bag. Shake and turn the bag to evenly coat wings.

3. Place wings skin-side up on the rack. Bake for 30 minutes, flip the wings over, and bake for an additional 20–30 minutes until wings are crispy and golden brown.

4. In a small saucepan, add hot sauce, buttery spread, and honey. Cook over medium heat for 1–2 minutes, stirring until ingredients are melted and combined. In a small bowl, combine cornstarch and water. Immediately add the cornstarch mixture to sauce and whisk to combine. Constantly whisk and cook sauce for 15–30 seconds until thickened.

5. Pour sauce into a large bowl. Immediately transfer hot wings to the large bowl and toss with sauce to coat.

Fried Green Tomatoes

Ingredients :

TOMATOES
- 3 large firm green tomatoes
- 1 teaspoon salt
- ½ cup unsweetened almond milk
- 1½ teaspoons white vinegar
- 1½ cups vegetable oil
- ½ cup gluten-free all-purpose flour with xanthan gum
- 1 cup gluten-free cornmeal
- ½ cup cornstarch
- 1 tablespoon seasoned salt

REMOULADE SAUCE
- 1 cup mayonnaise
- 1 teaspoon horseradish sauce
- ½ teaspoon onion powder
- ½ teaspoon paprika
- ¼ teaspoon garlic powder
- 1 teaspoon lemon juice
- ¼ teaspoon salt

Directions :

1. Slice tomatoes 1/4" thick and place on a paper towel–lined plate. Salt tomatoes on both sides and let sit for 10 minutes. (Do not skip this step; it helps draw extra water out of tomatoes so they are

crispier when fried.)

2. Add milk and vinegar into a pie pan or shallow dish and allow to sit for 1–2 minutes. Add tomatoes to the milk mixture.

3. Combine all the remoulade ingredients in a small bowl. Cover and refrigerate until serving.

4. Continue with tomatoes by heating oil in a large skillet over medium-high heat.

5. Combine flour, cornmeal, cornstarch, and seasoned salt to a pie pan or shallow dish. Mix until fully combined.

6. Dip milk-covered tomatoes into the flour mixture. Cover both sides of tomatoes with the mixture.

7. Place tomatoes into the skillet in batches of four or five. Do not crowd tomatoes; they should not touch each other. Cook 2 minutes on each side or until golden brown. Remove from pan and place on a paper towel–lined plate. Repeat with remaining tomatoes. Serve with remoulade sauce while tomatoes are still hot.

Avocado Spring Rolls with Cashew and Cilantro Dipping Sauce

Ingredients :

DIPPING SAUCE
- 4 teaspoons white vinegar
- 1 teaspoon balsamic vinegar
- ½ cup honey
- ½ cup chopped cashews
- 1¼ cups chopped fresh cilantro
- 1 tablespoon jarred minced garlic
- 2 green onions, sliced
- 1 tablespoon granulated sugar
- 1 teaspoon ground cumin
- ½ teaspoon ground turmeric
- ¼ cup olive oil

FILLING
- 2 large avocados, peeled, pitted, and diced
- ½ cup chopped sun-dried tomatoes packed in oil
- ¼ teaspoon chopped fresh cilantro

WRAPPING
- 8 (8") round rice paper wrappers
- 2 cups vegetable oil

Directions :

1. In a medium microwave-safe bowl, stir together vinegars and honey and microwave for 1 minute.
2. In a food processor purée cashews, 1 cup cilantro, garlic, onions, sugar, cumin, and turmeric.
3. Add the cashew mixture to the vinegar mixture and stir to combine. Add olive oil and stir to fully combine. Cover and refrigerate.
4. In a medium bowl, stir together the filling ingredients.
5. Fill a 9" cake pan with warm water. Submerge a rice paper into the water for 2 seconds. Place the rice papers on a cutting board, smooth-side down.
6. Place 2 tablespoons filling in the center of a paper. Fold the left and right edges of the rice paper in, then starting from the bottom, roll up to cover the filling. Then keep rolling until you reach the end. The rice paper is sticky, so it will seal itself. Place on a plate and repeat with remaining rice paper wrappers.
7. Heat oil in a large work or skillet over medium-high heat. Fry spring rolls in batches of four at a time for 2 minutes on each side until lightly golden. Remove with a slotted spoon to a paper towel–lined plate to absorb excess oil. Serve with dipping sauce.

Smoked Salmon Dip

Ingredients :
- 8 ounces dairy-free cream cheese
- ½ teaspoon horseradish sauce
- 2 tablespoons dried dill
- ½ teaspoon jarred minced garlic
- 1 tablespoon lemon juice
- ¼ teaspoon salt
- 1 tablespoon capers, minced
- 1 green onion, sliced
- 8 ounces smoked salmon

Directions :

1. Add all ingredients to the bowl of a food processor and pulse until salmon is chopped well and everything is combined. Do not overprocess.
2. Place dip in a small bowl, cover with plastic wrap, and refrigerator for at least 30 minutes before serving.

Easy Guacamole

- **Ingredients :**

- 3 large ripe avocados, peeled, pitted, and mashed
- 2 tablespoons lime juice
- ½ teaspoon salt
- ½ teaspoon ground cumin
- ½ medium sweet onion, peeled and diced
- 2 large Roma tomatoes, diced
- ½ cup chopped fresh cilantro
- ½ teaspoon jarred minced garlic

Directions :

1. In a large bowl, stir together avocado and lime juice and toss to coat. Add salt and cumin and stir to combine. Fold in onions, tomatoes, cilantro, and garlic and stir to fully combine ingredients.

Deep-Dish Pizza Bites

Ingredients :
- 2 large eggs, whisked
- ½ teaspoon garlic powder
- 1 teaspoon dried basil
- 1 teaspoon dried oregano
- 1⅓ cups Bisquick Gluten Free Pancake & Baking Mix
- ½ cup water
- ⅓ cup olive oil
- 1½ cups shredded dairy-free mozzarella cheese, divided
- ¾ cup gluten-free pizza sauce

Directions :

1. Preheat oven to 425°F. Spray a twelve-cup muffin tin with gluten-free nonstick cooking spray.

2. In a medium bowl, add eggs, garlic powder, basil, and oregano and stir until fully combined. Add Bisquick, water, and olive oil and mix well.

3. Fill each muffin well three-quarters full. Sprinkle 1 tablespoon dairy-free cheese over the top of batter. Spoon 1 tablespoon pizza sauce over cheese. Add another layer of cheese over sauce. Bake for 15 minutes. Allow to cool for 2 minutes before removing from pan.

Spinach, Sundried Tomatoes, and Artichoke Dip

Ingredients :
- 1 (10-ounce) package frozen chopped spinach, defrosted and drained
- 2 (13.75-ounce) cans artichoke hearts, drained and chopped
- 1 cup chopped sun-dried tomatoes
- ½ cup mayonnaise

- 8 ounces dairy-free cream cheese
- 1 tablespoon lemon juice
- ½ teaspoon jarred minced garlic
- ½ teaspoon onion powder

Directions :

1. Squeeze the excess liquid out of spinach. Add all ingredients to the bowl of a food processor and pulse until spinach and artichokes are chopped well and everything is combined. Do not overprocess.
2. Place dip in a small bowl, cover with plastic wrap, and refrigerator for at least 30 minutes before serving.

Sticky Asian Wings

Ingredients :

MARINADE
- ½ cup gluten-free soy sauce
- ½ cup lime juice
- 2 teaspoons jarred minced garlic
- 2 teaspoons jarred minced ginger
- 2 pounds chicken wingettes and drumettes

WING SAUCE
- ½ cup gluten-free apricot jam
- ½ teaspoon salt
- ⅛ teaspoon garlic powder
- 1 teaspoon jarred minced ginger
- ⅛ teaspoon onion powder
- ¼ cup lime juice

Directions :

1. In a large sealable plastic bag, add the marinade ingredients, seal, and turn the bag a few times to coat wings. Refrigerate overnight, turning occasionally. Before cooking, drain and discard marinade.
2. Preheat oven to 375°F.
3. Line a 9" x 13" baking pan with aluminum foil. Spray a baking rack with gluten-free nonstick cooking spray and place into pan. Place wings on the rack and bake for 15 minutes.
4. In a medium saucepan, combine the wing sauce ingredients. Stir to fully combine. Cook over medium heat and bring to a low boil. Simmer for 2 minutes.
5. Remove wings from oven and baste with sauce.
6. Bake for an additional 40 minutes, turning and basting wings every 10 minutes.

7. Take wings out of the oven and turn the oven to broil. Broil wings for 2–5 minutes until lightly charred.

Loaded Mashed Potato Bites

Ingredients :
- 3 cups cold mashed potatoes
- 4 strips gluten-free bacon, cooked and chopped
- 1 cup shredded dairy-free Cheddar cheese
- 1 green onion, sliced
- 2 large eggs, whisked
- 1½ cups gluten-free panko bread crumbs
- 2 cups vegetable oil

Directions :

1. In a large bowl, mix together mashed potatoes, bacon, cheese, and green onion.

2. Using a small cookie scoop, scoop out the potato mixture and roll into 1½" balls. Dip balls into eggs and then dredge in panko, pressing to coat on all sides.

3. Heat oil in a large skillet over medium-high heat. Working in batches, add balls to hot oil and cook for 2–3 minutes on each side until golden and crispy. Transfer to a paper towel–lined plate. Allow to cool for 2–4 minutes before serving.

Party Meatballs

Ingredients :

MEATBALLS
- ½ cup gluten-free bread crumbs
- 1 tablespoon Italian seasoning
- ½ tablespoon onion powder
- ½ teaspoon salt
- 1 tablespoon jarred minced garlic
- 6 tablespoons unsweetened almond milk
- 1 pound 90/10 ground beef
- 1 large egg, beaten

SAUCE
- 2 (12-ounce) bottles chili sauce
- 1 (32-ounce) jar gluten-free grape jelly

Directions :

1. Spray a slow cooker with gluten-free nonstick cooking spray.
2. Combine all the meatball ingredients in a large bowl. Use a cookie scoop or rounded tablespoon to form twenty-four meatballs. Place uncooked meatballs in the bottom of the slow cooker.
3. In a medium bowl, whisk together chili sauce and grape jelly. Pour over meatballs and cook on high for 3–4 hours until meatballs reach an internal temperature of 165°F.

Buffalo Chicken Dip

Ingredients :
- 2 (13-ounce) cans chicken breast, drained
- ½ cup mayonnaise
- ½ cup gluten-free and dairy-free ranch dressing
- 2 tablespoons gluten-free and dairy-free hot sauce

Directions :

1. Preheat oven to 350°F and spray an 8" × 8" casserole dish with gluten-free nonstick cooking spray.
2. In a large bowl, add chicken, using a fork to shred it into small pieces. Add mayonnaise, ranch dressing, and hot sauce and stir to combine.
3. Transfer to prepared baking dish and bake for 20 minutes. Allow to cool for 5 minutes before serving.

Southwestern Queso Dip

Ingredients :
- 1 cup cashews
- 1 cup unsweetened cashew milk
- ¼ cup nutritional yeast
- 1 tablespoon olive oil
- 2 (15-ounce) cans black beans, drained and rinsed
- 1½ cups gluten-free chunky salsa
- 2 tablespoons gluten-free taco seasoning

Directions :

1. Add water to a small saucepan and boil raw cashews in water for 5–10 minutes. Remove from heat and let cool in water, then drain. Blend in a food processor or blender with milk and yeast until smooth, scraping sides as needed.
2. Add the olive oil to a large skillet over medium heat. Add black beans, salsa, and taco seasoning and cook for 5–8 minutes, stirring until heated through. Stir in cashew sauce and stir to combine. Cook for 2–3 more minutes until thickened. Serve while hot.

Buffalo Chicken Bites

Ingredients :
- 1 (12.5-ounce) can chicken breast, drained
- ½ cup gluten-free and dairy-free buffalo wing sauce, divided
- ½ cup gluten-free and dairy-free ranch dressing, divided
- 2 cups shredded dairy-free Cheddar cheese
- 1½ cups Bisquick Gluten-Free Pancake & Baking Mix
- ¾ cup unsweetened almond milk

Directions :

1. Preheat oven to 350°F degrees. Line a baking sheet with parchment paper.

2. In a large bowl, add chicken, ¼ cup buffalo wing sauce, and ¼ cup ranch dressing. Stir to fully coat chicken.

3. Add cheese and Bisquick to the chicken mixture. Mix until fully combined. Add milk and mix until fully combined.

4. Using a cookie scoop or a rounded tablespoon, make approximately thirty-six 1" balls from the mixture. Place balls on prepared baking sheet. Bake for 22–26 minutes until golden brown. Serve with remaining ¼ cup buffalo wing sauce and ¼ cup ranch dressing for dipping.

Chili Lime Bacon-Wrapped Shrimp

- **Ingredients :**
- ¼ cup light brown sugar, packed
- 1 teaspoon onion powder
- 1 tablespoon jarred minced garlic
- ½ teaspoon chili powder
- 1 teaspoon paprika
- ¼ teaspoon kosher salt
- 2 tablespoons lime juice
- 2 tablespoons olive oil
- 20 large shrimp, peeled and deveined
- 10 strips gluten-free bacon, cut in half

Directions :

1. Combine all of the ingredients except shrimp and bacon in a sealable plastic bag. Add shrimp, seal the bag, and turn over several times so marinade covers shrimp. Place in the refrigerator for 30 minutes.

2. Preheat oven to 450°F and line a jelly roll pan with aluminum foil and spray with gluten-free nonstick cooking spray.

3. Wrap each shrimp with half slice bacon, securing with a toothpick.
4. Bake for 10–15 minutes until bacon is crisp and shrimp turn pink.

Fried Pickles

Ingredients :
- ½ cup unsweetened almond milk
- 1½ teaspoons white vinegar
- 2 cups sliced dill pickles, drained
- ½ cup gluten-free all-purpose flour with xanthan gum
- ½ cup gluten-free cornstarch
- 1 tablespoon seasoned salt
- 1½ cups vegetable oil

Directions :
1. Add milk and vinegar to a pie pan or shallow dish and allow to sit for 1–2 minutes. Add pickles to the milk mixture.
2. Combine flour, cornstarch, and salt to a separate pie pan or shallow dish. Mix until fully combined.
3. Dip milk-covered pickles into the flour mixture. Cover both sides of pickles with the mixture. Place on a plate.
4. Heat oil in a large skillet over medium-high heat.
5. Place pickles into the skillet in batches and fry for 1–2 minutes until golden brown; remove with a slotted spoon and drain on a paper towel–lined plate. Repeat with remaining pickles.

Mexican Street Corn Dip

Ingredients :
- 8 ounces dairy-free cream cheese, softened
- ½ cup mayonnaise
- 1 teaspoon jarred minced garlic
- ½ teaspoon chili powder
- ½ teaspoon ground cumin
- 2 tablespoons lime juice
- 2 (15-ounce) cans corn, drained
- 2 tablespoons peeled and chopped red onion
- ½ cup chopped fresh cilantro
- ¼ teaspoon paprika

Directions :
1. In a medium bowl, combine cream cheese, mayonnaise, garlic, chili powder, cumin, and lime juice

and mix until fully combined and smooth.

2. Add corn, onions, and cilantro and stir to combine. Cover and refrigerate for at least 30 minutes before serving. Sprinkle with paprika before serving.

Easy Homemade Hummus

Ingredients :
- ¼ cup tahini
- ¼ cup lemon juice
- 3 tablespoons olive oil, divided
- 2 teaspoons jarred minced garlic
- 1 teaspoon salt
- ½ teaspoon ground cumin
- 1 (15-ounce) can chickpeas, drained, divided

Directions :

1. Add tahini and lemon juice to the bowl of a food processor and process for 1 minute.

2. Add 2 tablespoons olive oil, garlic, salt, and cumin to the mixture and process for 1 minute. Add half of chickpeas to the food processor and process for 1 minute. Scrape sides and bottom of the bowl, then add remaining chickpeas and process for 1–2 minutes until thick and smooth.

3. Transfer hummus to a small bowl and drizzle with remaining 1 tablespoon olive oil.

Seven-Layer Dip

Ingredients :

DAIRY-FREE SOUR CREAM
- 6 ounces dairy-free plain Greek yogurt
- 1 teaspoon lemon juice

DIP
- 2 tablespoons gluten-free taco seasoning
- 1 (16-ounce) can gluten-free refried beans
- 2 cups guacamole
- 1 cup gluten-free salsa
- 1 cup shredded lettuce
- 1 cup dairy-free Cheddar cheese shreds
- ¼ cup sliced black olives
- ½ cup diced green onion
- ½ cup chopped fresh cilantro

- 1 (11-ounce) bag gluten-free tortilla chips

Directions :

1. Drain off any excess liquid from yogurt. Stir yogurt and lemon juice together in a small bowl. Cover and refrigerate at least 30 minutes before using.

2. In a small bowl, mix together sour cream and taco seasoning.

3. Spread beans onto the bottom of an 8" × 8" casserole dish sprayed with gluten-free nonstick cooking spray. Spread a layer of sour cream mixture over beans, then guacamole over the sour cream mixture, followed by a layer of salsa, then lettuce and cheese. Sprinkle olives, green onions, and cilantro over the top. Cover and refrigerate for 1 hour before serving. Serve with gluten-free tortilla chips.

Southwestern Spring Rolls

Ingredients :

FILLING
- ½ cup chopped cooked chicken
- 1 large avocado, peeled, pitted, and diced
- ¼ cup canned corn, drained and rinsed
- ¼ cup canned black beans, drained and rinsed
- ¼ cup chopped fresh cilantro
- 1 teaspoon ground cumin
- 2 teaspoons lime juice

WRAPPING
- 8 (8") round rice paper wrappers
- 2 cups vegetable oil

Directions :

1. In a medium bowl, stir together the filling ingredients.

2. Fill a 9" cake pan with warm water. Submerge a rice paper into the water for 2 seconds. Place the rice paper on a cutting board with smooth-side down.

3. Place 2 tablespoons filling in the center of the paper. Fold the left and right edges of the rice paper in, then starting from the bottom, roll up to cover the filling. Then keep rolling until you reach the end. The rice paper is sticky, so it will seal itself. Place on a plate and repeat with remaining rice paper wrappers.

4. Heat oil in a large work or skillet over medium-high heat. Fry spring rolls in batches of four at a time for 2 minutes on each side until lightly golden. Remove with a slotted spoon to a paper towel–lined plate to absorb excess oil and repeat with remaining rolls.

Thai Chicken Skewers with Peanut Sauce

Ingredients :

MARINADE
- 1 tablespoon gluten-free soy sauce
- 3 tablespoons lime juice
- ¼ teaspoon salt
- ⅛ teaspoon ground black pepper
- 1 tablespoon jarred minced garlic
- 1 tablespoon jarred minced ginger
- ½ teaspoon coriander
- ½ teaspoon ground cumin
- ½ teaspoon ground turmeric
- 2 tablespoons olive oil
- 2 pounds chicken tenders
- ¼ cup chopped fresh cilantro

DIPPING SAUCE
- 1 teaspoon jarred minced ginger
- ½ teaspoon jarred minced garlic
- ½ cup gluten-free peanut butter
- 2 teaspoons sesame oil
- 2 tablespoons gluten-free soy sauce
- 2 tablespoons lime juice
- 2 tablespoons light brown sugar, packed
- ¼ teaspoon sriracha
- ⅓ cup coconut milk beverage

Directions :

1. In a medium bowl, whisk together soy sauce, lime juice, salt, pepper, garlic, ginger, coriander, cumin, turmeric, and olive oil. Add chicken and toss with marinade, cover, and refrigerate for 30 minutes.

2. Preheat grill. Skewer chicken tenders. Grill chicken for 4–5 minutes on each side until it is browned on both sides and cooked through. Sprinkle with cilantro.

3. Combine the dipping sauce ingredients in a small bowl until smooth and serve on the side.

Italian Bruschetta

Ingredients :
- 8 large ripe Roma tomatoes, diced

- 6 fresh basil leaves, chopped
- ¼ teaspoon salt
- ⅛ teaspoon ground black pepper
- 2 tablespoons jarred minced garlic
- 4 tablespoons extra-virgin olive oil, divided
- 1 teaspoon balsamic vinegar
- 1 baguette gluten-free and dairy-free French bread

Directions :

1. In a medium bowl, combine tomatoes, basil, salt, pepper, garlic, 1 tablespoon olive oil, and balsamic vinegar. Cover and refrigerate for 30 minutes.
2. Preheat oven to broil. Slice baguette, brush with remaining olive oil, and place on a baking sheet and broil for 1–2 minutes until bread is toasted. Top with the tomato mixture and serve.

Smoked Salmon with Cucumber and Dill

Ingredients :
- 4 ounces dairy-free cream cheese, softened
- 2 tablespoons dried dill
- 2 tablespoons lemon juice
- 1 large English cucumber
- 4 ounces thinly sliced smoked salmon
- ½ teaspoon everything bagel seasoning

Directions :

1. In a medium bowl, mix together cream cheese, dill, and lemon juice until smooth.
2. With a vegetable peeler, stripe cucumber, leaving a small strip of skin in between each peel. Slice cucumber into ¼" slices.
3. Place cucumber slices on a platter. Place ½ teaspoon cream cheese mixture on each cucumber. Fold strips of smoked salmon and place on top of the mixture. Sprinkle with everything bagel seasoning before serving.

Classic Deviled Eggs

Ingredients :
- 6 large hard-boiled eggs, peeled and sliced in half, divided
- 2 tablespoons mayonnaise
- ½ teaspoon ground mustard
- ½ teaspoon white vinegar
- ¼ teaspoon salt
- ½ teaspoon dried dill

Directions :

1. Remove yolks and place in a small bowl. Mash yolks with a fork and stir in mayonnaise, mustard, vinegar, and salt.

2. Fill egg whites evenly with the yolk mixture. Sprinkle with dill. Cover and chill in the refrigerator for at least 30 minutes before serving.

Pico de Gallo

Ingredients :
- 12 large Roma tomatoes, chopped
- 1 cup peeled and chopped red onion
- 2 cups chopped fresh cilantro
- 1 small jalapeño pepper, veins and seeds removed, diced
- 3 tablespoons lime juice
- ½ teaspoon salt

Combine tomatoes, onions, cilantro, jalapeño, lime juice and salt in a small bowl. Cover and refrigerate for 30 minutes before serving.

Stuffed Mushrooms

Ingredients :
- 1 tablespoon olive oil
- ¼ cup peeled and finely chopped sweet onion
- ½ teaspoon jarred minced garlic
- 1 pound gluten-free ground sausage
- 1 tablespoon dried sage
- 8 ounces dairy-free cream cheese
- 3 tablespoons nutritional yeast
- ⅓ cup gluten-free bread crumbs
- 3 teaspoons dried basil
- 1 teaspoon dried parsley
- 30 large fresh baby bella mushrooms, stems removed
- 3 tablespoons dairy-free buttery spread, melted

Directions :

1. Preheat oven to 400°F. Spray a 9" × 13" baking dish with gluten-free nonstick cooking spray.

2. Heat olive oil in a large skillet over medium-high heat. Add onions and garlic and sauté for 30 seconds until garlic is fragrant. Add sausage and sage and cook for 6–8 minutes until sausage is no longer pink and onions are tender. Break up sausage into crumbles and drain. Add cream cheese and

nutritional yeast; cook and stir until melted. Stir in bread crumbs, basil, and parsley.

3. Place mushroom caps in prepared baking pan, stem-side up. Brush with buttery spread. Spoon the sausage mixture into mushroom caps. Bake uncovered for 12–15 minutes until mushrooms are tender.

Pressure Cooker Mexican Rice

Ingredients :
- 2 tablespoons olive oil
- ¼ cup peeled and chopped sweet onion
- 1 teaspoon jarred minced garlic
- 2 cups long-grain white rice
- 2½ cups gluten-free chicken broth
- ¾ cup canned crushed tomatoes, including liquid
- ½ teaspoon ground cumin
- ½ teaspoon chili powder
- ½ teaspoon paprika
- 1 teaspoon salt
- ½ cup chopped fresh cilantro, divided

Directions :

1. Set the pressure cooker to Sauté mode. When the display reads "Hot," add in olive oil, onions, and garlic. Sauté for 2–3 minutes or until garlic and onions are tender.

2. Add rice and stir until coated. Add in broth, tomatoes, cumin, chili powder, paprika, salt, and cilantro.

3. Press the Cancel button and place the lid on your pressure cooker and twist it so it locks in place and set the steam release knob to the Sealing position. Press the Manual button and set to 8 minutes. When the cooking cycle has finished, allow the pressure cooker to naturally release for 5 minutes. Once the pressure cooker reads "5 minutes," manually release by turning the knob to Venting. Hot steam will be released from the valve in venting mode. Once all steam has been released and the pressure valve lowers, remove the lid and serve. Take a fork and lightly fluff rice. Sprinkle with cilantro. Serve warm.

Pressure Cooker Collard Greens

Ingredients :
- 1 tablespoon olive oil
- 8 strips thick-cut gluten-free bacon, sliced
- ½ cup peeled and diced sweet onion
- 2 teaspoons jarred minced garlic

- 2 cups gluten-free chicken broth
- 1 tablespoon apple cider vinegar
- 1 tablespoon light brown sugar, packed
- 2 teaspoons seasoned salt
- 1 (16-ounce) bag chopped collard greens

Directions :

1. Set the pressure cooker to the Sauté setting. When the display reads "Hot," add olive oil. Add bacon, onions, and garlic and cook for 3–5 minutes, stirring occasionally, until tender.

2. Press the Cancel button. Add broth, vinegar, brown sugar, and salt; stir to combine. Add collard greens and put the lid on the pot and lock it into place. Set the steam release knob to the Sealing position. Press the Meat/Stew button and set to 35 minutes.

3. When the cooking cycle has finished, wait 10 minutes and then manually release the remaining steam by turning the knob to Venting. Hot steam will be released from the valve in venting mode. Once all steam has been released and the pressure valve lowers, remove the lid and serve. Serve warm.

Slow Cooker Black Beans

Ingredients :
- 1 pound dry black beans, picked over and rinsed
- 1 sweet onion, peeled and diced
- 2 teaspoons jarred minced garlic
- 1 bay leaf
- 2 teaspoons salt
- 6 cups water

Directions :

1. Place black beans, onions, garlic, bay leaf and salt in a slow cooker. Add water. Cover and cook on high for about 3–4 hours until beans are soft, testing after 3 hours. If cooking on low, set it for 6–8 hours until beans are soft, testing after 6 hours.

2. Remove bay leaf and allow beans to cool for 10 minutes before serving.

Slow Cooker Apples and Cinnamon

Ingredients :
- 5 large Granny Smith apples, peeled and sliced into ½"-thick slices
- 2 tablespoons dairy-free buttery spread, melted
- 1 tablespoon fresh lemon juice
- 6 tablespoons light brown sugar, packed
- 1 teaspoon ground cinnamon

- 2 tablespoons apple cider

Directions :

1. Spray a slow cooker with gluten-free nonstick cooking spray. Add apples, buttery spread, and lemon juice to the slow cooker and stir.

2. Sprinkle with brown sugar and cinnamon; toss to coat. Pour cider over apples. Cover and cook on low heat setting 3½ hours or until apples are tender.

Slow Cooker Pork Roast with Savory Gravy

Ingredients :
- 2 pounds pork loin roast
- ½ teaspoon salt
- ⅛ teaspoon ground black pepper
- 2 tablespoons olive oil
- ½ medium sweet onion, peeled and diced
- 2 tablespoons jarred minced garlic
- ½ cup gluten-free chicken broth
- 2 tablespoons gluten-free Worcestershire sauce
- 2 teaspoons dried thyme
- 1 teaspoon dried rosemary
- 1 tablespoon cornstarch
- 3 tablespoons water

Directions :

1. Season pork with salt and pepper. Set the pressure cooker to the Sauté setting and add olive oil. Add pork and sear the sides a golden brown. Add onions and garlic and cook for 2 minutes until soft.

2. In a small bowl, stir together broth, Worcestershire sauce, thyme, and rosemary. Pour over pork. Press the Cancel button and put the lid on the pot and lock it into place. Set the steam release knob to the Sealing position. Press the Manual button and set to 30 minutes. When the cooking cycle has finished, manually release by turning the knob to Venting. Hot steam will be released from the valve in venting mode. Once all steam has been released and the pressure valve lowers, remove the lid and check that internal temperature of pork is 145°F.

3. Remove pork from the pressure cooker, place on a cutting board, cover with aluminum foil and allow to rest for 10 minutes.

4. Mix together cornstarch and water. Add to the pressure cooker with the juices. Turn pressure cooker on to Sauté and simmer until thickened. Slice pork, place on plates, and drizzle with gravy.

Pressure Cooker Baked Potatoes

Ingredients :
- 1 cup water
- 4 medium russet potatoes

Directions :

1. Place the metal trivet inside of the pressure cooker and add water.

2. Poke potatoes with a fork several times all over. Place potatoes on top of the wire rack. Place lid on pressure cooker and lock it into place. Set the steam release knob to the Sealing position. Press the Manual button and set to 14 minutes.

3. When the cooking cycle has finished, let it naturally release for 10 minutes, and then manually release by turning the knob to Venting. Hot steam will be released from the valve in venting mode. Once all steam has been released and the pressure valve lowers, remove the lid and serve.

Pressure Cooker Mashed Potatoes

Ingredients :
- 7 medium russet potatoes, peeled
- 4 cups water
- ⅓ cup dairy-free buttery spread
- ¼ cup unsweetened almond milk
- 2 teaspoons salt

Directions :

1. Add potatoes to the cooker and pour water over them. Place lid on the pressure cooker and lock it into place. Set the steam release knob to the Sealing position. Press the Manual button and set to 12 minutes.

2. When the cooking cycle has finished, manually release pressure. Once all steam has been released and the pressure valve lowers, remove the lid and drain.

3. Transfer potatoes to a large bowl. Add buttery spread, milk, and salt and mash with a potato masher until you reach desired texture and smoothness.

Pressure Cooker New Orleans–Style Red Beans and Rice

Ingredients :
- 2 tablespoons olive oil
- 1 pound gluten-free andouille sausage, sliced
- 1 cup peeled and chopped sweet onion
- 1 cup seeded and chopped green bell pepper
- 1 cup chopped celery
- 1 tablespoon jarred minced garlic

- 1 teaspoon dried thyme
- 2 teaspoons Cajun seasoning
- 4 cups gluten-free chicken broth
- 2 bay leaves
- 1 pound small red beans, soaked overnight or quick-soaked and drained
- 1 smoked ham hock
- 4 cups cooked white rice
- 2 green onions, sliced
- ¼ cup chopped fresh parsley

Directions :

1. Set the pressure cooker to the Sauté mode and add olive oil. Add sausage and cook for 5 minutes until browned. Remove with a slotted spoon to plate and set aside.

2. Add onions, bell peppers, celery, and garlic. Cook for 5 minutes until onion is translucent. Stir in thyme and Cajun seasoning. Stir in broth, bay leaves, red beans, and ham hock.

3. Press the Cancel button and place the lid on pressure cooker and lock it into place. Set the steam release knob to the Sealing position. Press the Manual button and set to 30 minutes. Allow to completely release pressure naturally (15–30 minutes). Once all steam has been released and the pressure valve lowers, remove the lid and remove the ham hock, chop into bite-sized pieces, and return back to the pot. Remove bay leaves. Add the sausage back into the pot and stir. Select Sauté mode and allow beans to thicken for 5 minutes. Serve over rice and garnish with green onions and parsley.

Pressure Cooker Whole Roasted Chicken

Ingredients :
- 1 teaspoon garlic powder
- 1 tablespoon onion powder
- 1 tablespoon dried oregano
- 1 tablespoon dried thyme
- 1 tablespoon dried sage
- 1 teaspoon salt
- 1 (4-pound) whole roasting chicken, innards removed
- 1 medium lemon, halved
- 2 tablespoons olive oil
- 1 cup gluten-free chicken broth

Directions :

1. In a small bowl, combine seasonings. Dry chicken skin with paper towels. Rub the seasoning mixture all over chicken, including the cavity. Place lemons into the cavity.

2. Set the pressure cooker to the Sauté setting. Add olive oil and chicken, breast-side down, and cook

for 4 minutes until golden brown. Using tongs, turn chicken over and cook for 4 minutes. Remove chicken and set aside.

3. Place a metal trivet into the pot and add broth. Place chicken on top of the trivet. Place lid on pressure cooker and lock it into place. Set the steam release knob to the Sealing position. Press the Manual button and set to 28 minutes. Allow to completely pressure release naturally (15–30 minutes). Once all steam has been released and pressure valve has lowered, remove the lid and let rest for 10–15 minutes. Serve immediately.

Pressure Cooker Hard-Boiled Eggs

Ingredients :
- 1 cup water
- 6 large eggs

Directions :

1. Place water in the pressure cooker. Add in an egg or steam rack and carefully set eggs as desired.

2. Place lid on pressure cooker and lock it into place. Set the steam release knob to the Sealing position. Press the Manual button and set to 5 minutes.

3. When the cooking cycle has finished, let pressure release naturally for 5 minutes, then manually release by turning the knob to Venting. Hot steam will be released from the valve in venting mode. Once all steam has been released and pressure valve has lowered, remove the lid. Carefully remove eggs from pressure cooker and place in a large bowl of ice water. Let eggs sit in water bath for 5 minutes. Remove eggs from water bath. Crack eggs and peel.

Pressure Cooker Cashew Chicken

Ingredients :
- 2 tablespoons sesame oil, divided
- ½ cup gluten-free soy sauce
- 3 tablespoons rice wine vinegar
- 3 tablespoons ketchup
- 1 tablespoon honey
- 1 tablespoon jarred minced garlic
- 1 tablespoon jarred minced ginger
- ½ teaspoon Chinese five-spice powder
- ¼ teaspoon crushed red pepper flakes
- 1 pound boneless, skinless chicken breasts, cut into 1" pieces
- 3 tablespoons gluten-free cornstarch, divided
- ¼ teaspoon salt
- ¼ teaspoon ground black pepper

- 2 tablespoons water
- 1 cup chopped cashews
- 4 cups cooked rice
- 1 green onion, sliced

Directions :

1. To make the sauce: in a medium bowl, whisk together 1 tablespoon oil, soy sauce, vinegar, ketchup, honey, garlic, ginger, five-spice powder, and red pepper flakes and set aside.

2. Add chicken to a sealable plastic bag. Pour in 2 tablespoons cornstarch, salt, and black pepper. Seal top and turn the bag several times to coat chicken.

3. Add remaining 1 tablespoon oil to the pressure cooker and turn it on to Sauté. Allow oil to heat up for 1 minute and then add coated chicken. Sear for 2 minutes.

4. Press the Cancel button and pour sauce into the pressure cooker. Stir to coat chicken with sauce. Place lid on pressure cooker and lock it into place. Set the steam release knob to the Sealing position. Press the Manual button and set to 10 minutes.

5. In a small bowl, stir to combine remaining 1 tablespoon cornstarch with water until cornstarch is dissolved.

6. When the cooking cycle has finished, manually release by turning the knob to Venting. Hot steam will be released from the valve in venting mode. Once all steam has been released and pressure valve has lowered, remove the lid. Press the Sauté button and pour the cornstarch mixture into the pressure cooker and whisk into sauce. Add cashews and continue stirring for 1–2 minutes until sauce has thickened. Serve over rice and sprinkle with green onions.

Pressure Cooker Steak Sandwich

Ingredients :
- 1 pound rib eye steak
- ½ teaspoon salt
- ½ teaspoon garlic powder
- 1 teaspoon dried thyme
- ½ teaspoon dried oregano
- 2 tablespoons olive oil
- 1 large green bell pepper, seeded and sliced
- 1 large red bell pepper, seeded and sliced
- 1 cup sliced mushrooms
- 1 large sweet onion, peeled and sliced
- 1 tablespoon gluten-free Worcestershire sauce
- ½ cup gluten-free beef broth

Directions :

1. Freeze steak for 30 minutes. Cut steak against the grain into very thin strips and set aside.

2. In a small bowl, add salt, garlic powder, thyme, and oregano. Stir to combine. Sprinkle on steak strips.

3. Set the pressure cooker to the Sauté setting and add olive oil. Sauté bell peppers, mushrooms, and onions for 5 minutes. Add the seasoned beef strips on top of sautéed vegetables.

4. In a small bowl, mix together Worcestershire sauce and beef broth. Pour the mixture over the meat and vegetables.

5. Place lid on the pressure cooker and lock it into place. Set the steam release knob to the Sealing position. Press the Manual button and set to 8 minutes.

6. When the cooking cycle has finished, let pressure release naturally for 12 minutes, then manually release by turning the knob to Venting. Hot steam will be released from the valve in venting mode. Once all steam has been released and pressure valve has lowered, remove the lid. Save broth to serve as au jus for dipping. Serve with the rolls.

Slow Cooker Southern-Style Pinto Beans

Ingredients :
- 1 pound dry pinto beans, rinsed, picked over for tiny stones and soaked 6–8 hours or overnight
- 1 teaspoon chili powder
- ½ teaspoon dried oregano
- 1 tablespoon seasoned salt
- 1 teaspoon olive oil
- 3 slices pork fatback, chopped
- 4 cups water
- 1 small sweet onion, peeled and chopped

Directions :

1. Add beans to a slow cooker and stir in chili powder, oregano, and salt.

2. Add olive oil to a large skillet and heat over medium-high heat. Add fat back to the skillet and cook for 2 minutes. Place meat and any rendered fat in the slow cooker with beans.

3. Pour water into slow cooker and add onions. Stir well to combine, place lid on and cook on high for 5 hours until beans are very tender.

Pressure Cooker Sweet Potatoes

Ingredients :
- 4 medium sweet potatoes
- 1½ cups water

Directions :

1. Add a steaming trivet to the pressure cooker, place potatoes on top of the trivet, and pour in water.
2. Place lid on the pressure cooker and lock it into place. Set the steam release knob to the Sealing position. Press the Manual button and set to 18 minutes.
3. When the cooking cycle has finished, let pressure release naturally, about 15 minutes. Once all steam has been released and the pressure valve lowers, remove the lid and serve potatoes.

Texas-Style Slow Cooker Beef Chili

Ingredients :
- 1 tablespoon olive oil
- 1 teaspoon minced fresh garlic
- 1 large sweet onion, peeled and diced
- 2 large green bell peppers, seeded and diced
- 1 pound 90/10 ground beef
- 1 (4-ounce) can diced green chile peppers
- 1¾ cups gluten-free beef broth
- 1 (15-ounce) can pinto beans, drained and rinsed
- 1 (14-ounce) can diced tomatoes, including liquid
- 2 (8-ounce) cans tomato sauce
- 1 (6-ounce) can tomato paste
- 1 tablespoon ground cumin
- 2 tablespoons chili powder
- 1 teaspoon dried oregano
- 1 tablespoon light brown sugar, packed
- 1 teaspoon salt
- ¼ teaspoon ground black pepper

Directions :

1. Heat olive oil in a large skillet over medium-high heat. Add garlic, onions, and green peppers and sauté for 2–5 minutes until vegetables are softened. Add beef and cook for 5–8 minutes until no longer pink; drain.
2. Add the beef mixture to a slow cooker. Add remaining ingredients and stir well to combine. Place top on the slow cooker and cook on low for 4–6 hours.

Rotisserie-Style Shredded Chicken

Ingredients :

CHICKEN
- 2 tablespoons olive oil

- 4 (6-ounce) boneless, skinless chicken breasts

ROTISSERIE SEASONING
- 1 tablespoon dried sage
- 1 tablespoon dried thyme
- 1 tablespoon onion powder
- 1 tablespoon dried oregano
- 1 teaspoon garlic powder
- 1 teaspoon salt

PRESSURE COOKER
- 1 cup gluten-free chicken broth

SLOW COOKER
- 2 cups gluten-free chicken broth

Directions :

For either appliance:

1. Add olive oil and chicken to the pot. Add all the rotisserie seasoning ingredients to a medium bowl and stir to combine. Pour broth into the bowl with the seasoning mix and stir. Pour seasoned chicken broth over chicken.

For the pressure cooker:

1. Place lid on the pressure cooker and lock it into place. Set the steam release knob to the Sealing position. Press the Manual button and set to 12 minutes. When the cooking cycle has finished, let pressure release naturally for 10 minutes, then manually release by turning the knob to Venting. Hot steam will be released from the valve in venting mode. Once all steam has been released and pressure valve has lowered, remove the lid. Check that internal temperature of chicken is 165°F. Shred chicken with remaining liquid in the pot.

For the slow cooker:

1. Cook on low 6–8 hours or on high 3–4 hours until the internal temperature reaches 165°F. Once the cook time is over, turn the slow cooker off. Pour half of the liquid out of the pot and shred chicken with remaining liquid in the pot. (The slow cooker version contains a bit more salt, 470mg, than the pressure cooker version.)

Pressure Cooker Barbecue Pulled Pork

Ingredients :
- 1 tablespoon light brown sugar, packed
- 1 tablespoon garlic powder
- 1 tablespoon onion powder

- 1 tablespoon chili powder
- 1 tablespoon salt
- 1 tablespoon paprika
- 1 tablespoon ground cumin
- 1 teaspoon mustard powder
- 1 (3-pound) boneless pork roast, cut into 2" cubes
- 1 tablespoon olive oil
- 1 cup gluten-free chicken broth
- 1 tablespoon apple cider vinegar
- 2 cups gluten-free barbecue sauce, divided

Directions :

1. In a large bowl, combine brown sugar and all spices. Add in pork and toss to coat with the spice mixture.

2. Add olive oil to the pressure cooker and turn on to Sauté. Add pork pieces in a single layer. Brown on all sides, then transfer to a plate and set aside. Repeat with remaining pieces of pork. Press Cancel to turn the cooker off.

3. Add the broth, vinegar, and 1 cup barbecue sauce to cooker and stir to combine. Add in pork and stir to coat with the sauce mixture. Place lid on pressure cooker and lock it into place. Set the steam release knob to the Sealing position. Press the Manual button and set to 60 minutes.

4. When the cooking cycle has finished, let pressure naturally release. Once all steam has been released and pressure valve has lowered, remove the lid.

5. Transfer pork to a separate clean plate with a slotted spoon, leaving juices behind. Turn on to Sauté once more and let sauce simmer for 10 minutes until it has thickened and reduced by more than half. Shred pork with two forks.

6. Once sauce has reduced, skim the fat off the top with a spoon and discard. Add shredded pork and remaining 1 cup barbecue sauce into the cooker and toss to coat with sauce. Serve immediately.

Pressure Cooker Chicken Cacciatore

Ingredients :
- 4 (4-ounce) bone-in, skin-on chicken thighs
- 1 teaspoon salt
- ⅛ teaspoon ground black pepper
- 2 tablespoons olive oil
- 1 tablespoon jarred minced garlic
- 1 small sweet onion, peeled and diced
- 1 large green bell pepper, seeded and diced
- 1 cup sliced mushrooms
- 1 cup diced celery

- 1 (14-ounce) can stewed tomatoes
- 3 tablespoons tomato paste
- 2 tablespoons Italian seasoning
- ¾ cup gluten-free chicken broth

Directions :

1. Season chicken with salt and pepper. Set the pressure cooker to the Sauté setting and add olive oil. Add chicken and cook until browned, about 6 minutes per side. Transfer chicken to a plate.

2. Place garlic, onions, peppers, mushrooms, and celery in the pot; cook for 5 minutes until soft. Place chicken back in the pot; add tomatoes and tomato paste. Sprinkle with Italian seasoning and pour in chicken broth. Place lid on the pressure cooker and lock it into place. Set the steam release knob to the Sealing position. Press the Manual button and set to 11 minutes.

3. When the cooking cycle has finished, manually release pressure. Once all steam has been released and the pressure valve lowers, remove the lid and check chicken for doneness; an instant-read thermometer inserted near the bone should read 165°F. Serve.

Pressure Cooker Corned Beef and Cabbage

Ingredients :
- 1 small yellow onion, peeled and sliced
- 2 teaspoons jarred minced garlic
- Pickling spice packet from corned beef
- 3 cups water
- 1 (4–pound) corned beef brisket, rinsed
- 1 pound tiny potatoes
- 1 pound baby carrots
- 1 head cabbage, cut into 8 wedges

Directions :

1. Place a metal trivet inside of the pressure cooker. Add onions, garlic, pickling spices, and water in the cooker. Place corned beef brisket, fat-side up, on a rack on top of onions. Place lid on pressure cooker and lock it into place. Set the steam release knob to the Sealing position. Press the Manual button and set to 85 minutes.

2. When the cooking cycle has finished, let pressure naturally release for 20 minutes, then manually release the remaining pressure. Once all steam has been released and pressure valve has lowered, remove the lid. Remove corned beef to a cutting board and cover with aluminum foil to keep warm.

3. Strain cooking liquid into a small bowl and discard solids. Return 1½ cups liquid to the cooker and reserve remaining liquid. Add potatoes, carrots, and cabbage to the cooker. Place lid on pressure cooker and lock it into place. Set the steam release knob to the Sealing position. Press the Manual

button and set to 4 minutes. Manually release pressure. Once all steam has been released and pressure valve has lowered, remove the lid.

4. Slice corned beef against the grain. Spoon reserved cooking liquid over corned beef slices. Remove vegetables from the cooker with a slotted spoon and serve with corned beef.

Slow Cooker Beef Tips and Gravy

Ingredients :
- 3 tablespoons olive oil, divided
- 3 pounds top sirloin, cubed
- 1 teaspoon seasoned salt
- ⅛ teaspoon fresh ground black pepper
- 1 cup peeled and diced sweet onion
- 2 tablespoons jarred minced garlic
- 1 cup sliced mushrooms
- 2 cups gluten-free beef broth
- 1 tablespoon gluten-free Worcestershire sauce
- 2 teaspoons Italian seasoning
- 1 teaspoon dried thyme
- 2 tablespoons cornstarch
- 3 tablespoons water

Directions :

1. Heat 1 tablespoon olive oil in a large skillet over medium-high heat. Add beef, sprinkle with salt and pepper and cook for 2–4 minutes until seared on each side. Add 2 tablespoons of olive oil to the bottom of the slow cooker. Remove beef to slow cooker and top with onions, garlic, and mushrooms.

2. Add beef broth and Worcestershire sauce to the slow cooker and sprinkle beef with Italian seasoning and thyme.

3. Cover and cook on low for 6–7 hours or on high for 3–4 hours until beef is tender.

4. Whisk together cornstarch and water in a small bowl and add to slow cooker. Stir until sauce has thickened and cook on low for an additional 10 minutes before serving.

Pressure Cooker Indian Butter Chicken

Ingredients :
- 4 tablespoons dairy-free buttery spread
- 1 cup peeled and chopped sweet onion
- 3 tablespoons jarred minced garlic
- 2 tablespoons jarred minced ginger
- 1 tablespoon curry powder

- 2 teaspoons garam masala
- 1 teaspoon salt
- ¾ teaspoon smoked paprika
- 2 pounds boneless, skinless chicken thighs cut into 1" pieces
- 1 (15-ounce) can tomato sauce
- 1 cup full-fat unsweetened canned coconut milk
- ¼ cup chopped fresh cilantro

Directions :

1. Add the buttery spread, onions, garlic, ginger, and all spices in the pressure cooker. Turn pressure cooker on to Sauté for 5 minutes, stirring occasionally. Press the Cancel button.
2. Add chicken and tomato sauce. Place lid on pressure cooker and lock it into place. Set the steam release knob to the Sealing position. Press the Manual button and set to 7 minutes.
3. When the cooking cycle has finished, manually release pressure by turning the knob to Venting. Hot steam will be released from the valve in venting mode. Once all steam has been released and pressure valve has lowered, remove the lid.
4. Stir in milk. Turn the pressure cooker on to Sauté again and simmer for 2 minutes to thicken sauce. Serve topped with cilantro.

Slow Cooker Pot Roast with Savory Gravy

Ingredients :
- 1 tablespoon olive oil
- 1 teaspoon salt
- 1 (3-pound) chuck roast
- 2 cups baby carrots
- 1 cup sliced celery
- 1 cup halved baby potatoes
- 1 tablespoon onion powder
- 1 tablespoon dried sage
- 1 tablespoon dried thyme
- 1 teaspoon dried rosemary
- 1 teaspoon dried garlic powder
- 1 tablespoon apple cider vinegar
- 1 cup gluten-free beef broth
- 1 tablespoon cornstarch
- 1 tablespoon gluten-free all-purpose flour with xanthan gum

Directions :

1. Add olive oil into a slow cooker. Salt beef roast and add to slow cooker. Add the carrots, celery, and potatoes.

2. In a small bowl, combine seasonings, vinegar, and broth and stir to combine. Pour the beef broth mixture over vegetables and beef.

3. Cook on high for 4–5 hours until vegetables and meat are tender. Using a slotted spoon, remove beef and vegetables to a platter and cover with aluminum foil to keep warm.

4. Pour liquid from the slow cooker into a small saucepan. Add cornstarch and flour and whisk over medium heat until fully combined. Bring to a slight boil, stirring until thickened. Remove the roast from the slow cooker and place on a cutting board to be sliced. Serve with gravy.

Pressure Cooker Chicken, Broccoli, and Rice

Ingredients :
- 2 tablespoons olive oil
- 1 tablespoon jarred minced garlic
- 3 (6-ounce) boneless, skinless chicken breasts, cut into 1" cubes
- 1½ cups uncooked white rice
- 1⅓ cups gluten-free chicken broth
- 1 tablespoon gluten-free Worcestershire sauce
- ½ teaspoon salt
- ¼ teaspoon ground black pepper
- 1 teaspoon dried thyme
- 2 tablespoons onion powder
- 1 tablespoon lemon juice
- 3 cups unsweetened almond milk
- 3 tablespoons gluten-free all-purpose flour with xanthan gum
- 1 cup frozen broccoli florets

Directions :

1. Add olive oil to pressure cooker and turn on to Sauté. Add garlic and chicken and cook for 1 minute, stirring occasionally so chicken gets browned on both sides.

2. Add rice, broth, Worcestershire sauce, salt, pepper, thyme, onion powder, lemon juice, and stir to combine. Place lid on cooker and lock it into place. Set the steam release knob to the Sealing position. Press the Manual button and set to 5 minutes.

3. In a small bowl, whisk together milk and flour and set aside.

4. When the cooking cycle has finished, manually release pressure by turning the knob to Venting. Hot steam will be released from the valve in venting mode. Once all steam has been released, remove the lid. Immediately add the milk mixture and mix until well combined.

5. Add the broccoli and place lid back on cooker and lock it in place. Set the steam release knob to the sealing position. Press the Manual button and set to 5 minutes. When the cooking cycle has finished, manually release pressure by turning the knob to Venting. Hot steam will be released from the valve

in venting mode. Once all steam has been released, remove the lid, stir, and serve.

Slow Cooker Lemon Garlic Chicken

Ingredients :
- 4 cups quartered red potatoes
- ½ cup peeled and diced sweet yellow onion
- 1 cup peeled and sliced carrots
- 1 tablespoon jarred minced garlic
- 6 (4-ounce) bone-in, skin-on chicken thighs
- ½ teaspoon salt
- ¼ teaspoon ground black pepper
- ¼ cup olive oil
- ¼ cup lemon juice
- ½ teaspoon dried rosemary
- 1 teaspoon dried thyme
- 1 lemon, sliced

Directions :

1. Place potatoes, onions, carrots, and garlic in the bottom of a slow cooker.

2. Sprinkle chicken thighs with salt and pepper and place in slow cooker. Pour olive oil evenly over top, followed by lemon juice, rosemary, and thyme. Place lemon slices over top.

3. Cook on high for 4 hours or on low for 8 hours. When chicken is finished cooking, remove and place on a baking sheet greased with gluten-free nonstick cooking spray. Preheat oven to broil and place baking sheet under the broiler for 3–4 minutes until chicken is browned and crisp. Remove lemon slices from the cooker and squeeze over chicken. Serve chicken with vegetables.

Slow Cooker Orange Chicken

Ingredients :
- ¼ cup cornstarch
- 1 teaspoon salt
- ¼ teaspoon ground black pepper
- 3 (6-ounce) boneless, skinless chicken breasts, cut into 1" pieces
- ¼ cup vegetable oil
- ¾ cup orange marmalade
- ¼ cup gluten-free soy sauce
- 1 tablespoon rice vinegar
- 1 teaspoon sesame oil
- 1 teaspoon jarred minced garlic
- 1 teaspoon jarred minced ginger

- 1 tablespoon sesame seeds
- 2 tablespoons sliced green onion

Directions :

1. Add cornstarch, salt, and pepper to a sealable plastic bag. Add chicken to the bag and seal. Turn bag over several times to coat chicken.

2. Heat vegetable oil in a large skillet over medium-high heat. Add chicken in a single layer and cook for 3–4 minutes on each side until browned, working in batches.

3. Coat a slow cooker with gluten-free nonstick cooking spray and add chicken.

4. In a small bowl, whisk together orange marmalade, soy sauce, vinegar, sesame oil, garlic, and ginger. Pour sauce over chicken and gently stir to coat. Cook on low for 2–3 hours. Sprinkle with sesame seeds and green onions, then serve.

Chocolate Chip Cookies

Ingredients :
- 1 cup dairy-free buttery spread
- ¾ cup granulated sugar
- ¾ cup light brown sugar, packed
- 1 large egg
- 1 teaspoon molasses
- 1 teaspoon pure vanilla extract
- 2½ cups gluten-free all-purpose flour with xanthan gum
- ½ teaspoon baking soda
- ½ teaspoon gluten-free baking powder
- ½ teaspoon salt
- 2 cups gluten-free and dairy-free chocolate chips

Directions :

1. Preheat oven to 375°F and line two baking sheets with parchment paper.

2. In a large bowl, beat buttery spread, granulated sugar, and brown sugar at medium speed until smooth and creamy.

3. Add egg, molasses, and vanilla extract and mix until fully combined.

4. In a medium bowl, stir together flour, baking soda, baking powder, and salt and stir to combine. Add the flour mixture to the buttery spread mixture and mix until fully combined. Add chocolate chips and mix on low until chips are fully combined.

5. Scoop batter with a greased 1½-tablespoons cookie scoop and place cookies 2" apart on prepared baking sheet.

6. Bake for 8–10 minutes until cookies start to turn golden brown. Allow to cool for 2–3 minutes

before moving to a cooling rack. Store in an airtight container at room temperature for up to 3 days.

Fluffy Sugar Cookies

Ingredients :
- ¾ cup dairy-free buttery spread
- ¾ cup granulated sugar
- 1 large egg
- 1 tablespoon pure vanilla extract
- ⅛ teaspoon pure almond extract
- 1½ cups gluten-free all-purpose flour with xanthan gum
- 1 teaspoon gluten-free baking powder
- ⅛ teaspoon salt

Directions :

1. Preheat oven to 375°F and line two baking sheets with parchment paper.
2. In a large bowl, beat buttery spread and sugar together on medium speed until smooth.
3. Beat in egg, vanilla extract, and almond extract.
4. In a small bowl, stir together flour, baking powder, and salt.
5. Slowly pour the flour mixture into batter and mix until fully combined.
6. Scoop batter with a greased 1½-tablespoons cookie scoop and place cookies 2" apart on a prepared baking sheet. Bake for 10–12 minutes or until the edges are very lightly browned. Allow cookies to cool for 2–3 minutes before moving to a cooling rack. Store in an airtight container at room temperature for up to 3 days.

The Perfect Pie Crust

Ingredients :
- ¼ cup dairy-free buttery spread, diced
- ¼ cup shortening
- 3 tablespoons ice-cold water
- 1¼ cups gluten-free all-purpose flour with xanthan gum
- 2 tablespoons granulated sugar
- ¼ teaspoon salt
- 1 large egg
- ¼ teaspoon apple cider vinegar

Directions :

1. Put buttery spread, shortening, and water in separate small bowls. Put the bowls in the freezer for about 5 minutes.

2. Add remaining ingredients in the bowl of a stand-up mixer and mix with the paddle attachment until all ingredients are fully combined. (To make the pie crust if you do not have a mixer, cut buttery spread into flour, sugar and salt and then add the rest of the ingredients, mixing and forming into a ball.)

3. Shape dough into a ball, wrap in plastic wrap, and refrigerate at least 1 hour.

4. Remove from the refrigerator and let stand at room temperature for 15 minutes. Spay a 9" pie pan with gluten-free nonstick cooking spray.

5. Unwrap dough and place onto lightly floured parchment paper. Sprinkle dough with flour; top with plastic wrap or another sheet of parchment paper.

6. Use a rolling pin to roll dough out into a circle. Peel the plastic wrap or parchment paper off the top of dough circle.

7. Carefully place crust into prepared pie pan. Press dough into the bottom and sides (lift pie crust up and do not try to stretch it). Seal any cracks, if necessary. Fill and bake as directed in your pie recipe.

Butter Pound Cake

Ingredients :

CAKE
- 1 cup unsweetened almond milk
- 1 tablespoon white vinegar
- 1 cup dairy-free buttery spread
- 2 cups granulated sugar
- 4 large eggs
- 1 tablespoon pure vanilla extract
- 3 cups gluten-free all-purpose flour with xanthan gum
- 1 teaspoon gluten-free baking powder
- ½ teaspoon baking soda

GLAZE
- ⅓ cup dairy-free buttery spread, melted
- ¾ cup sugar
- 2 tablespoons water
- 2 teaspoons pure vanilla extract

Directions :

1. Preheat oven to 325°F and spray a Bundt pan with gluten-free nonstick cooking spray.

2. In a small bowl, add milk and vinegar and allow to sit for 5 minutes to make buttermilk.

3. In a large bowl, beat buttery spread and sugar together on medium speed until smooth.

4. Add remaining cake ingredients to large bowl and mix until fully combined. The batter will be very thick. Pour batter into prepared Bundt pan and bake for 70 minutes or until a toothpick inserted in the center comes out clean.

5. Combine the glaze ingredients in a small saucepan over medium-low heat. Stir continuously until buttery spread is melted and sugar is dissolved, 2–3 minutes. Do not bring to a boil.

6. Poke holes all over warm cake with a knife and pour glaze evenly over cake while still in the pan. Allow cake to cool completely in the pan and then invert cake onto a serving plate. Store in an airtight container at room temperature for up to 3 days.

Fudgy Brownies

Ingredients :
- ½ cup dairy-free buttery spread, melted
- 1 tablespoon pure vanilla extract
- ¾ cup granulated sugar
- ½ cup light brown sugar, packed
- 2 large eggs, room temperature
- ¾ cup gluten-free all-purpose flour with xanthan gum
- ½ cup cocoa powder
- ½ teaspoon baking soda
- ½ teaspoon salt

Directions :

1. Preheat oven to 350°F and line an 8" × 8" baking pan with parchment paper and coat the bottom and sides with gluten-free nonstick cooking spray or buttery spread.

2. In a large bowl, add buttery spread, vanilla extract, granulated sugar, and brown sugar and mix until fully combined.

3. Add in eggs one at a time and mix until fully combined.

4. In a medium bowl, stir together flour, cocoa powder, baking soda, and salt.

5. Slowly add the flour mixture to the buttery spread mixture and mix until fully combined and smooth.

6. Pour brownie batter into prepared baking pan. Bake for 30–35 minutes or until a toothpick inserted in the center comes out just barely clean and the sides of brownies start to pull away from the pan. Let brownies cool completely, about 30 minutes, in the pan before slicing. Store in an airtight container at room temperature for up to 3 days.

Classic Vanilla Cake with Chocolate Buttercream

Ingredients :

CAKE
- ⅔ cup dairy-free buttery spread
- 1½ cups granulated sugar
- 3 large eggs
- 1 tablespoon pure vanilla extract
- 2¼ cups gluten-free all-purpose flour with xanthan gum
- 3½ teaspoons gluten-free baking powder
- ½ teaspoon salt
- 1½ cups unsweetened almond milk

CHOCOLATE BUTTERCREAM FROSTING
- 1 cup dairy-free buttery spread
- 2 teaspoons pure vanilla extract
- ¼ teaspoon pure almond extract
- 1 cup cocoa powder
- ⅛ teaspoon salt
- 4 cups confectioners' sugar
- 3 tablespoons milk

Directions :

1. Preheat oven to 350°F and spray two 9" round cake pans with gluten-free nonstick cooking spray.

2. In a large bowl, cream together buttery spread and sugar until smooth. Add eggs and vanilla extract and mix until fully combined.

3. Add flour, baking powder, and salt and mix until combined. Pour in milk and mix for 2 minutes on medium until batter is smooth.

4. Pour batter into prepared cake pans. Bake for 30–35 minutes or until a toothpick inserted in the center comes out clean. Cool in pans for 10 minutes and then remove from the pans and transfer to a wire rack to finish cooling, about 10–15 minutes. Allow cake to completely cool before frosting.

5. In a large bowl, cream buttery spread until smooth. Add vanilla and almond extracts and mix until fully combined. Add cocoa powder and salt and mix until fully combined. Add the confectioners' sugar 1 cup at a time and mix until fully combined. Add milk and beat until smooth and spreadable. Spread frosting between layers of cake and cover the top and sides. Store in an airtight container at room temperature for up to 3 days.

Cinnamon Roll Cake

Ingredients :

CAKE

- 3 cups gluten-free all-purpose flour with xanthan gum
- ¼ teaspoon salt
- 1 cup granulated sugar
- 4 teaspoons gluten-free baking powder
- 1½ cups unsweetened almond milk
- 2 large eggs
- 2 teaspoons pure vanilla extract
- ½ cup dairy-free buttery spread, melted

TOPPING
- 1 cup dairy-free buttery spread, softened
- 1 cup light brown sugar, packed
- 2 tablespoons gluten-free all-purpose flour with xanthan gum
- 1 tablespoon ground cinnamon

GLAZE
- 2 cups confectioners' sugar
- 5 tablespoons unsweetened almond milk
- 1 teaspoon pure vanilla extract

Directions :

1. Preheat oven to 350°F and spray a 9" × 13" glass baking pan with gluten-free nonstick cooking spray.
2. In a large bowl, add flour, salt, sugar, baking powder, milk, eggs, and vanilla and mix until fully combined. Add buttery spread and mix until fully combined. The cake batter will be very thick and sticky. Pour into prepared baking pan.
3. In a medium bowl, beat together the topping ingredients until smooth.
4. Drop tablespoons of topping into cake batter and use a knife to swirl it around.
5. Bake at 350°F for 35–40 minutes or until a toothpick inserted in the center comes out clean.
6. In a separate medium bowl, mix together the glaze ingredients until smooth. Pour over warm cake and serve. Store in an airtight container at room temperature for up to 3 days.

Pumpkin Bread Cookies

Ingredients :

COOKIES
- 1 teaspoon baking soda
- 1 cup canned pumpkin
- ½ cup dairy-free buttery spread

- 1 cup sugar
- 1 large egg, room temperature
- 1 teaspoon pure vanilla extract
- 2 cups gluten-free all-purpose flour with xanthan gum
- ¼ teaspoon salt
- 1 tablespoon pumpkin pie spice
- 1 teaspoon ground cinnamon

GLAZE
- ½ cup confectioners' sugar
- 1 teaspoon pure vanilla extract
- ¼ teaspoon pumpkin pie spice
- 4 tablespoons pure maple syrup
- 1 teaspoon unsweetened almond milk

Directions :

1. Preheat oven to 350°F and line two baking sheets with parchment paper.
2. In a small bowl, stir together baking soda and canned pumpkin and set aside for 2 minutes.
3. In a large bowl, beat buttery spread and sugar together on medium speed until smooth. Add egg and beat until the mixture is light and fluffy. Add the pumpkin mixture and vanilla extract into the buttery spread mixture and mix until fully combined.
4. In a medium bowl, stir together flour, salt, and spices. Pour the flour mixture into the pumpkin mixture and mix until fully combined. The cookie batter will be thick.
5. Scoop batter with a greased 1½-tablespoons cookie scoop and place cookies 2" apart on prepared baking sheets.
6. Bake for 15–20 minutes or until bottoms of cookies are lightly golden brown.
7. Combine the glaze ingredients in a small bowl and stir until smooth. Drizzle over warm cookies. Store cookies in an airtight container at room temperature for up to 3 days.

Apple Bundt Cake

Ingredients :

CAKE
- 1 cup unsweetened almond milk
- 1 tablespoon white vinegar
- 1 cup dairy-free buttery spread
- 2 cups granulated sugar
- 4 large eggs

- 1 tablespoon pure vanilla extract
- 3 cups gluten-free all-purpose flour with xanthan gum
- 1 teaspoon gluten-free baking powder
- ½ teaspoon baking soda
- 1 tablespoon ground cinnamon
- 3 cups peeled and chopped Gala apples
- 1 cup chopped pecans

GLAZE
- ⅓ cup dairy-free buttery spread, melted
- ¾ cup light brown sugar, packed
- 2 tablespoons water
- 2 teaspoons pure vanilla extract
- ¼ teaspoon ground cinnamon

Directions :

1. Preheat oven to 325°F. Spray a Bundt pan with gluten-free nonstick cooking spray.

2. Add milk and vinegar to a small bowl and allow to sit for 5 minutes to make buttermilk.

3. In a large bowl, beat buttery spread and sugar together on medium speed until smooth. Add eggs and vanilla extract and mix until combined. Add flour, baking powder, baking soda, and cinnamon and mix until fully combined. Add the milk mixture and stir until fully combined. The batter will be very thick. Stir in apples and pecans.

4. Pour batter into prepared Bundt pan and bake for 70 minutes or until a toothpick inserted in the center comes out clean.

5. Combine the glaze ingredients in a small saucepan over medium-low heat. Stir continuously until buttery spread is melted and brown sugar is dissolved, 2–3 minutes. Do not bring to a boil.

6. Poke holes all over warm cake with a knife and pour glaze evenly over cake while still in the pan.

7. Allow cake to cool completely in the pan and then invert cake onto a serving plate. Store in an airtight container at room temperature for up to 3 days.

Peanut Butter Cookies

- **Ingredients :**
- ½ cup plus 1 tablespoon granulated sugar, divided
- ½ cup light brown sugar, packed
- ½ cup dairy-free buttery spread, softened
- ½ cup gluten-free peanut butter
- 1 large egg
- 1 teaspoon molasses
- 1¼ cups plus 1 tablespoon gluten-free all-purpose flour with xanthan gum, divided

- ¾ teaspoon baking soda
- ½ teaspoon gluten-free baking powder

Directions :

1. Add ½ cup granulated sugar, brown sugar, buttery spread, and peanut butter in a large bowl and mix with a mixer at medium speed until fully combined and creamy.

2. Mix in egg and molasses until fully combined.

3. In a medium bowl, stir together flour, baking soda, and baking powder.

4. Slowly pour the flour mixture into the peanut butter mixture and mix until fully combined. The cookie dough will be like soft Play-Doh.

5. Cover cookie dough and refrigerate for 30 minutes.

6. Preheat oven to 375°F. Line two baking sheets with parchment paper.

7. Scoop 1 tablespoon of dough and roll into a ball. Place onto prepared baking sheets 2" apart.

8. Add remaining tablespoon flour into a small bowl. Dip the bottom of a fork into the flour and then press down on the tops of cookies to make a crisscross "x" shape. Sprinkle the tops of cookies with remaining sugar.

9. Bake for 10–12 minutes or until light brown on the edges. Allow cookies to cool for 3–5 minutes before moving to a cooling rack. Store in an airtight container at room temperature for up to 3 days.

Pineapple Upside Down Cake

Ingredients :

TOPPING
- ¼ cup dairy-free buttery spread, melted
- ⅔ cup light brown sugar, packed
- 1 (20-ounce) can sliced pineapple, drained
- 9 maraschino cherries, stems removed

CAKE
- ⅓ cup dairy-free buttery spread
- 1 cup sugar
- 1 teaspoon pure vanilla extract
- 1 large egg
- 1⅓ cups gluten-free all-purpose flour with xanthan gum
- 1½ teaspoons gluten-free baking powder
- ½ teaspoon salt
- 1 cup unsweetened almond milk

Directions :

1. Preheat oven to 350°F and spray a 9" × 9" pan with gluten-free nonstick cooking spray.
2. Pour melted buttery spread into the bottom of the pan. Sprinkle brown sugar over buttery spread. Place pineapple slices on top of brown sugar and then place a cherry in the center of each pineapple slice.
3. Cream buttery spread and sugar together. Add vanilla extract and egg and mix until fully combined.
4. Add flour, baking powder, and salt to the mixture and mix until fully combined. Pour in milk and mix for 2 minutes on medium speed until batter is smooth.
5. Pour cake batter over fruit in the cake pan. Bake for 50–55 minutes or until a toothpick inserted in the center comes out clean. Cool cake for 10 minutes, then invert cake onto a serving plate and serve warm. Store in an airtight container at room temperature for up to 3 days.

Carrot Cake with Cream Cheese Frosting

Ingredients :

CAKE
- 1½ cups applesauce
- 2 cups granulated sugar
- 3 large eggs
- 2 cups gluten-free all-purpose flour with xanthan gum
- 1 teaspoon baking soda
- ½ teaspoon gluten-free baking powder
- 2 teaspoons ground cinnamon
- ¼ teaspoon ground nutmeg
- ⅛ teaspoon ground cloves
- ¼ teaspoon ground allspice
- ½ teaspoon salt
- 2 cups peeled and grated carrots
- 1 cup shredded sweetened coconut
- 1 cup crushed pineapple in juice (not syrup), do not drain
- ½ cup raisins
- ½ cup chopped pecans
- 1 teaspoon pure vanilla extract

CREAM CHEESE FROSTING
- 1 cup dairy-free buttery spread, softened
- 2 (8-ounce) packages dairy-free cream cheese, softened
- 3 cups confectioners' sugar
- 2 tablespoons lemon juice
- 1 teaspoon pure vanilla extract

Directions :

1. Preheat oven to 350°F. Cut parchment paper for the bottom of two 8" cake pans and spray with gluten-free nonstick cooking spray.

2. In a large bowl, mix applesauce, sugar, and eggs until fully combined.

3. In a medium bowl, stir together flour, baking soda, baking powder, cinnamon, nutmeg, cloves, allspice, and salt. Stir in carrots, coconut, pineapple, raisins, pecans, and vanilla extract into the applesauce mixture. Add the flour mixture to batter and mix until fully combined. Divide batter equally between prepared cake pans.

4. Bake on the middle rack for 35–40 minutes or until a toothpick inserted in the center comes out clean and the sides of cakes are pulling away from the pans.

5. In a large bowl, beat buttery spread and cream cheese together on medium speed until smooth and creamy. Beat in confectioners' sugar 1 cup at a time. Beat in lemon juice and vanilla extract.

6. Cool cakes in the pans for about 10–15 minutes. Then use a knife to loosen cakes around the edges of the pans and invert cakes onto a cooling rack to completely cool before frosting. Spread frosting between layers of cake and cover top and sides. Store in an airtight container in the refrigerator for up to 3 days.

Better Than Banana Bread Cookies

- **Ingredients :**
- 3 large ripe bananas, peeled and mashed
- 1 teaspoon baking soda
- ½ cup dairy-free buttery spread
- 1 cup sugar
- 1 large egg
- 1 teaspoon pure vanilla extract
- 2 cups gluten-free all-purpose flour with xanthan gum
- ⅛ teaspoon salt
- ½ teaspoon ground cinnamon
- ¼ teaspoon ground nutmeg

Directions :

1. Preheat oven to 350°F and line two baking sheets with parchment paper.

2. In a medium bowl, mix together bananas and baking soda and let sit for 2 minutes.

3. In a large bowl, beat buttery spread and sugar together on medium speed until smooth. Add egg and vanilla extract and mix until the mixture is light and fluffy.

4. Add the banana mixture to the buttery spread mixture.

5. In a medium bowl, stir together flour, salt, and spices.

6. Pour the flour mixture into the banana mixture and mix until fully combined.

7. Scoop batter with a greased 1½-tablespoons cookie scoop and place cookies 2" apart on prepared baking sheets.

8. Bake for 11–13 minutes or until golden brown. Allow cookies to cool for 2–3 minutes before moving to cooling rack. Store in an airtight container at room temperature for up to 3 days.

Dutch Apple Pie

Ingredients :

FILLING
- 6 cups thinly sliced apples, such as Jazz apples
- 1 tablespoon lemon juice
- ⅔ cup granulated sugar
- ¼ cup gluten-free all-purpose flour with xanthan gum
- 1 tablespoon ground cinnamon
- ½ teaspoon ground nutmeg
- ⅛ teaspoon salt

PIE CRUST
- 1 (9") gluten-free and dairy-free pie crust (see The Perfect Pie Crust recipe in this chapter)

TOPPING
- 1 cup gluten-free all-purpose flour with xanthan gum
- ½ cup light brown sugar, packed
- ½ cup dairy-free buttery spread

Directions :

1. Preheat oven to 425°F.

2. Add apples to a large bowl and sprinkle with lemon juice and toss to coat apples.

3. In a small bowl, stir together sugar, flour, cinnamon, nutmeg, and salt. Sprinkle mixture over apples and toss until apple slices are evenly coated. Transfer apple mixture into pie crust.

4. In a medium bowl, combine the topping ingredients with a fork or pastry blender until the mixture resembles small crumbs. Sprinkle apple mixture with topping.

5. Place pie pan on a baking sheet. Cover the pie crust edge with a 3" aluminum foil strip, to prevent overbrowning. Bake on the middle rack for 40 minutes. Remove the foil from the crust and then cover the top of the pie loosely with aluminum foil and bake for an additional 10 minutes until pie crust and crumb topping are deep golden brown and filling begins to bubble. Transfer to a cooling

rack and allow pie to cool for 2–3 hours at room temperature before serving. Cover leftovers and keep at room temperature for 24 hours or refrigerated for up to 4 days.

Cowboy Cookies

Ingredients :
- 1½ cups gluten-free all-purpose flour with xanthan gum
- 1½ teaspoons gluten-free baking powder
- 1½ teaspoons baking soda
- 2 tablespoons ground cinnamon
- ½ teaspoon salt
- ¾ cup dairy-free buttery spread
- ¾ cup sugar
- ¾ cup light brown sugar, packed
- 2 large eggs
- 2 teaspoons pure vanilla extract
- 1½ cups gluten-free and dairy-free chocolate chips
- 1½ cups gluten-free quick oats
- 1 cup sweetened coconut shreds
- 1 cup chopped pecans

Directions :

1. Preheat oven to 350°F and line three baking sheets with parchment paper.
2. In a small bowl, mix together flour, baking powder, baking soda, cinnamon, and salt.
3. Add buttery spread to a large bowl and beat with a mixer at medium speed until smooth and creamy. Beat in sugars until combined. Add eggs, one at a time, and vanilla extract and beat until smooth.
4. Add the flour mixture and mix until fully combined. Add chocolate chips, oats, coconut, and pecans and mix until combined.
5. Using a greased 1½-tablespoons cookie scoop, place cookies 2" apart on prepared baking sheets.
6. Bake for 15–17 minutes until edges are lightly browned. Allow cookies to cool for 5 minutes before transferring to wire racks to cool further. Store in an airtight container at room temperature for up to 3 days.

Cinnamon Apple Fries

Ingredients :
- 4 Granny Smith apples, peeled and cut into sticks
- 1 tablespoon lemon juice
- 3 cups vegetable oil

- 1 cup cornstarch
- ½ teaspoon salt
- 1 teaspoon ground cinnamon
- 1 cup sugar

Directions :

1. In a large bowl, toss apples with lemon juice.
2. Heat oil in a large skillet over high heat.
3. Add cornstarch and salt to a large sealable plastic bag. Add apples to the bag, seal, and turn over and shake to coat apple slices.
4. Fry apple slices in oil for 2–3 minutes until golden brown.
5. Remove the fried apples from the skillet with a slotted spoon and place on a paper towel–lined plate to drain. Repeat with remaining apple slices.
6. In a large bowl, combine cinnamon and sugar. Toss apples in the mixture and serve warm.

White Cake with Almond Vanilla Buttercream

Ingredients :

CAKE
- ⅔ cup dairy-free buttery spread
- 1⅔ cups granulated sugar
- 1 teaspoon pure almond extract
- 2¼ cups gluten-free all-purpose flour with xanthan gum
- 3½ teaspoons gluten-free baking powder
- ½ teaspoon salt
- 1½ cups unsweetened almond milk
- 5 large egg whites

ALMOND VANILLA BUTTERCREAM
- 1 cup dairy-free buttery spread
- 1½ teaspoons pure vanilla extract
- ¼ teaspoon pure almond extract
- 4 cups confectioners' sugar

Directions :

1. Preheat oven to 350°F. Cut parchment paper for the bottom of two 8" cake pans and spray with gluten-free nonstick cooking spray.
2. In a large bowl, beat together buttery spread and sugar on medium speed until smooth. Add almond extract and mix to combine. Add flour, baking powder, and salt and mix until fully combined. Add

milk and mix until fully combined.

3. Beat in egg whites and mix on high for 2 minutes.
4. Divide the batter evenly between prepared cake pans.
5. Bake on the middle rack for 23–28 minutes or until a toothpick inserted in the center comes out clean and the sides of cakes are pulling away from the pans.
6. In a large bowl, beat buttery spread at medium speed until smooth. Add vanilla and almond extracts. Mix until fully combined.
7. Add confectioners' sugar 1 cup at a time and mix until combined.
8. Cool cakes in the pans for about 10–15 minutes. Then use a knife to loosen cakes around the edges of the pans and invert cakes onto a cooling rack to completely cool before frosting. Spread frosting between layers of cake and cover top and sides. Store in an airtight container for up to 3 days.

Strawberry Cupcakes with Strawberry Buttercream Frosting

Ingredients :

CUPCAKES
- ½ cup unsweetened almond milk
- 2 teaspoons white vinegar
- ¼ cup dairy-free buttery spread
- 1½ cups granulated sugar
- ½ teaspoon pure vanilla extract
- 3 large eggs
- 1½ cups gluten-free all-purpose flour with xanthan gum
- 1½ teaspoons gluten-free baking powder
- ½ teaspoon salt
- 1 cup strawberry purée

STRAWBERRY BUTTERCREAM FROSTING
- 1 cup dairy-free buttery spread, softened
- ½ cup strawberry purée
- ¼ teaspoon lemon juice
- ¼ teaspoon pure vanilla extract
- 3 cups confectioners' sugar

Directions :

1. Preheat oven to 350°F and line two twelve-cup cupcake tins with baking cup liners.
2. In a small bowl, combine milk and vinegar and allow to sit for 5 minutes to make buttermilk.

3. In a large bowl, beat buttery spread and sugar. Add vanilla. Add eggs one at a time to the mixture and mix until fully combined.

4. In a medium bowl, stir together flour, baking powder, and salt. Add the flour mixture to the buttery spread mixture. Mix until combined. Add strawberry purée and the milk mixture to batter. Mix until combined.

5. Scoop batter into prepared cupcake tins. Bake for 20 minutes or until a toothpick inserted in the center of a cupcake comes out clean. Remove cupcakes to a rack to cool. Allow to completely cool before frosting, about 30 minutes.

6. In a large bowl, beat buttery spread until smooth. Use a spatula to scrape down the sides of the bowl before adding the next ingredients.

7. Add strawberry purée, lemon juice, and vanilla extract and mix until fully combined. Use a spatula to scrape down the sides of the bowl before adding powdered sugar.

8. Add confectioners' sugar 1 cup at a time. Mix until frosting is firm. Refrigerate frosting for 5 minutes before either piping or spreading on top of cupcakes.

Lemon Crinkle Cookies

Ingredients :
- ¾ cup dairy-free buttery spread
- 1 cup sugar
- 1 teaspoon pure vanilla extract
- 1 large egg
- 1½ tablespoons lemon juice
- 1 teaspoon dried lemon peel
- 1¾ cups gluten-free all-purpose flour with xanthan gum
- ¼ teaspoon baking soda
- ½ teaspoon gluten-free baking powder
- ½ teaspoon salt
- ½ cup confectioners' sugar

Directions :

1. In a large bowl, beat buttery spread and sugar together on medium speed until smooth. Add vanilla extract, egg, lemon juice, and lemon peel and mix until fully combined.

2. Add flour, baking soda, baking powder, and salt and mix until fully combined.

3. Cover and refrigerate dough for 1 hour. Preheat oven to 350°F and line two baking sheets with parchment paper.

4. Add the confectioners' sugar to a small bowl. Scoop dough with a greased 1½-tablespoons cookie scoop and roll cookies in confectioners' sugar. Roll to cover all sides and place sugared dough balls 2" apart on prepared baking sheets.

5. Bake for 12–13 minutes until cookies start to turn golden brown. Allow cookies to cool for 5 minutes before moving to a cooling rack. Store in an airtight container in the room temperature for up to 3 days.

Double Chocolate Chip Cookies

Ingredients :
- ½ cup dairy-free buttery spread
- ¼ cup granulated sugar
- ¾ cup light brown sugar, packed
- 1 large egg, room temperature
- 1 tablespoon unsweetened almond milk
- 2 teaspoons pure vanilla extract
- 1½ cups gluten-free all-purpose flour with xanthan gum
- ¼ teaspoon salt
- ½ cup cocoa powder
- 1 teaspoon baking soda
- 1 cup gluten-free and dairy-free chocolate chips

Directions :

1. Preheat oven to 350°F degrees and line two baking sheets with parchment paper.

2. In a large bowl, beat buttery spread, granulated sugar, and brown sugar on medium speed until creamy.

3. Beat in egg, milk, and vanilla and mix until fully combined.

4. In a medium bowl, stir together flour, salt, cocoa powder, and baking soda.

5. Add the flour mixture to the buttery spread mixture and mix until fully combined. Add in chocolate chips and mix until fully combined.

6. Scoop cookie dough using a greased 1½-tablespoons cookie scoop and place cookies onto prepared baking sheets 2" apart. Bake for 11–12 minutes.

7. Allow cookies to cool on the baking sheet for at least 5 minutes before transferring to a wire rack to cool completely. Store in an airtight container at room temperature for 3 days.

Mini "Cheesecakes"

Ingredients :

FILLING
- 1½ cups cashews
- ⅔ cup full-fat unsweetened canned coconut milk, refrigerated

- ⅓ cup lemon juice
- ⅓ cup coconut oil, melted
- ⅓ cup pure maple syrup
- 1 teaspoon pure vanilla extract

CRUST
- 1 cup pecans
- 1 cup soft pitted dates, packed
- ¼ teaspoon pure vanilla extract
- ½ teaspoon ground cinnamon
- ⅛ teaspoon sea salt

Directions :

1. To prepare cashews for filling, add cashews to a medium heatproof bowl, cover with boiling water, and let them soak for 1 hour. Then drain.
2. Line two twelve-cup muffin tins with baking cup liners.
3. In a food processor, add the crust ingredients and process until the mixture resembles a loose dough. Press 1 tablespoon into the bottom of each muffin cup.
4. Scoop 2/3 cup off the top of the cold (and hardened) milk from the top of the can (leaving the clear liquid underneath) and add to a blender. Add soaked and drained cashews, lemon juice, coconut oil, maple syrup, and vanilla extract and blend together until very smooth.
5. Pour the cashew mixture over the crusts in the muffin tin. Cover with aluminum foil and place in the freezer for 2–3 hours to allow the mixture to set. When ready to serve, allow to thaw for 5 minutes at room temperature. Store leftovers in an airtight container in the refrigerator for up to 3 days.

Old-Fashioned Oatmeal Raisin Cookies

Ingredients :
- ½ cup dairy-free buttery spread
- ½ cup granulated sugar
- ½ cup light brown sugar, packed
- ½ teaspoon pure vanilla extract
- 1 large egg
- 1 cup gluten-free all-purpose flour with xanthan gum
- ½ teaspoon baking soda
- ½ teaspoon gluten-free baking powder
- ¼ teaspoon salt
- 1 teaspoon ground cinnamon
- 1½ cups gluten-free quick oats
- 1 cup raisins

Directions :

1. Preheat oven to 375°F. Line two baking sheets with parchment paper.
2. In a large bowl, beat together buttery spread, granulated sugar, and brown sugar on medium speed until smooth. Add vanilla extract and egg and mix until fully combined.
3. Add flour, baking soda, baking powder, salt, cinnamon, oats to the mixture and mix until fully combined. Mix in raisins until fully combined.
4. Scoop dough with a greased 1½-tablespoons cookie scoop and place cookies 2" apart on a parchment-lined baking sheet.
5. Bake for 10–12 minutes until cookies start to turn golden brown. Allow cookies to cool for 2–3 minutes before moving to a cooling rack. Store in an airtight container at room temperature for up to 3 days.

Apple Crisp

Ingredients :

TOPPING
- ½ cup gluten-free all-purpose flour with xanthan gum
- ½ cup gluten-free quick oats
- ½ cup light brown sugar, packed
- ½ teaspoon gluten-free baking powder
- ¼ teaspoon ground cinnamon
- ⅛ teaspoon salt
- ⅓ cup dairy-free buttery spread

FILLING
- 4 cups peeled and chopped Granny Smith apples
- 3 tablespoons dairy-free buttery spread, melted
- 2 tablespoons gluten-free all-purpose flour with xanthan gum
- 1 tablespoon lemon juice
- 3 tablespoons unsweetened almond milk
- 1 teaspoon pure vanilla extract
- ¼ cup light brown sugar, packed
- ½ teaspoon ground cinnamon
- ⅛ teaspoon salt

Directions :

1. Preheat oven to 375°F and spray an 8" × 8" baking pan with gluten-free nonstick cooking spray.
2. In a medium bowl, combine the topping ingredients with a fork or pastry blender until it resembles

small crumbs. Refrigerate while you prepare the filling.

3. Add apples to a large bowl.

4. In a small bowl, stir together buttery spread and flour until well blended. Add lemon juice, milk, and vanilla extract and stir to combine. Add brown sugar, cinnamon, and salt and stir until fully combined.

5. Pour the mixture over apples and toss to coat. Pour the apple mixture into prepared baking pan and spread into an even layer. Sprinkle topping evenly over apples. Bake for 30–35 minutes or until golden brown. Remove from the oven and cool for 10 minutes before serving.

Pistachio Cookies

Ingredients :
- ½ cup dairy-free buttery spread, softened
- ¾ cup light brown sugar, packed
- ¼ cup granulated sugar
- 1 box (3.5-ounce) gluten-free pistachio instant pudding
- 1 large egg
- 2 tablespoons unsweetened almond milk
- ½ teaspoon pure almond extract
- ½ teaspoon gluten-free green food coloring
- 1½ cups gluten-free all-purpose flour with xanthan gum
- ¼ teaspoon salt
- 1 teaspoon baking soda
- ½ cup finely chopped pistachios

Directions :

1. Preheat oven to 350°F degrees and line three baking sheets with parchment paper.

2. In a large bowl, beat buttery spread until creamy. Add brown sugar and granulated sugar and beat until creamy.

3. Beat in pudding mix, egg, milk, and almond extract until fully combined. Add green food coloring and mix until fully combined.

4. In a medium bowl, mix together flour, salt, and baking soda. Add the flour mixture to the buttery spread mixture and mix until fully combined. Add nuts and mix until fully combined.

5. Scoop cookie dough using a 1½-tablespoons cookie scoop, place cookies onto prepared baking sheets 2" apart, and bake for 10–12 minutes. Allow cookies to cool on the baking sheet for at least 5 minutes before transferring to a wire rack to cool completely. Store cookies in an airtight container at room temperature for up to 3 days.

Coconut Cream Pie

Ingredients :

CRUST
- 2 large egg whites
- 2⅔ cups shredded sweetened coconut
- 3 tablespoons dairy-free buttery spread, melted

FILLING
- ⅓ cup gluten-free all-purpose flour with xanthan gum
- ⅔ cup sugar
- 2 cups coconut milk beverage (carton)
- 2 large egg yolks
- 1 cup shredded sweetened coconut
- 1 tablespoon pure vanilla extract
- 1 teaspoon dairy-free buttery spread

TOPPING
- 1 (14-ounce can) coconut cream, refrigerated overnight
- 1 teaspoon pure vanilla extract
- ¾ cup confectioners' sugar
- 2 tablespoons cornstarch

Directions :

1. Preheat oven to 350°F and grease a 9" pie pan with gluten-free nonstick cooking spray.

2. In a large bowl, stir together egg whites, shredded coconut, and buttery spread. Pat the mixture into prepared pie pan to make crust. Bake crust for 20–25 minutes or until golden brown.

3. In a medium saucepan, mix together flour, sugar, milk, and egg yolks. Cook and stir over medium-high heat until mixture comes to a boil. Boil for only 1 minute. Remove from heat and add coconut, vanilla extract, and buttery spread. Pour custard filling into crust. Cover and refrigerate for 3 hours.

4. Chill a large bowl and whisk attachments of a mixer in the freezer for 10 minutes.

5. Scrape out the top of the chilled and thickened coconut cream (leaving the liquid behind) and place hardened coconut cream in chilled bowl. Beat for 30 seconds with mixer until creamy. Then add vanilla extract, confectioners' sugar, and cornstarch and mix for 1 minute until creamy and smooth. Use immediately or cover and refrigerate. Before serving pie, spread coconut whip on top of pie or on each individual slice. Store leftovers covered in the refrigerator for up to 3 days.

Hummingbird Cake with Cream Cheese Frosting

Ingredients :

CAKE
- ⅓ cup unsweetened almond milk
- 1 teaspoon white vinegar
- 1 cup dairy-free buttery spread
- 2 cups granulated sugar
- 4 large eggs
- 1 tablespoon pure vanilla extract
- 3 cups gluten-free all-purpose flour with xanthan gum
- ½ teaspoon gluten-free baking powder
- 1 teaspoon baking soda
- 1 teaspoon ground cinnamon
- 1 teaspoon salt
- 3 large ripe bananas, peeled and mashed
- 1 (8-ounce) can crushed pineapple, including liquid
- 1 cup chopped pecans

FROSTING
- 1 cup dairy-free buttery spread
- 2 (8-ounce) packages dairy-free cream cheese
- 2 tablespoons lemon juice
- 1 tablespoon pure vanilla extract
- 3 cups confectioners' sugar
- ½ cup chopped pecans

Directions :

1. Preheat oven to 350°F and spray two 9" round cake pans with gluten-free nonstick cooking spray.

2. In a small bowl, add milk and vinegar and allow to sit for 2–3 minutes to make buttermilk.

3. In a large bowl, cream together buttery spread and sugar until smooth. Add eggs one at a time and vanilla extract and mix until fully combined.

4. Add flour, baking powder, baking soda, cinnamon, and salt and mix until fully combined. Pour in the milk mixture and mix for 2 minutes on medium until batter is smooth. Add bananas, pineapple, and 1 cup pecans and mix until fully combined.

5. Divide batter evenly between the two cake pans. Bake for 30–35 minutes or until a toothpick inserted in the center comes out clean. Cool in pans for 10 minutes and then transfer to a wire rack to finish cooling, about 10–15 minutes.

6. In a large bowl, cream buttery spread and cream cheese together until smooth. Add lemon juice and vanilla extract and mix until fully combined. Add confectioners' sugar 1 cup at a time and beat until smooth and spreadable.

7. Allow cake to completely cool before frosting. Spread frosting between layers of cake and cover top and sides. Sprinkle the top of frosted cake with ½ cup chopped pecans.

Red Velvet Cookies

Ingredients :
- ½ cup dairy-free buttery spread, softened
- ¾ cup light brown sugar, packed
- ¼ cup granulated sugar
- 1 large egg
- 1 tablespoon unsweetened almond milk
- 2 teaspoons pure vanilla extract
- 1 tablespoon gluten-free red food coloring
- 1½ cups gluten-free all-purpose flour with xanthan gum
- ¼ teaspoon salt
- ¼ cup cocoa powder
- 1 teaspoon baking soda
- 1 cup gluten-free and dairy-free chocolate chips

Directions :
1. In a large bowl, beat buttery spread until creamy. Add brown sugar and granulated sugar and beat until creamy.
2. Beat in egg, milk, and vanilla extract and mix until fully combined. Add red food coloring and mix until fully combined.
3. In a medium bowl, mix together flour, salt, cocoa powder, and baking soda and whisk together until fully combined.
4. Add the flour mixture to the buttery spread mixture and mix until fully combined. Mix in chocolate chips until fully combined. Cover cookie dough and refrigerate for at least 1 hour.
5. Preheat oven to 350°F degrees and line two baking sheets with parchment paper.
6. Scoop cookie dough using a 1½-tablespoons cookie scoop and roll into twenty-four balls. Place cookie balls onto prepared baking sheets 2" apart and bake for 11–12 minutes. (The cookies will not spread too much while baking but you will flatten them next.)
7. Take cookies out of the oven and press down on warm cookies to slightly flatten. Allow cookies to cool on baking sheets for at least 5 minutes before transferring to a wire rack to cool completely. Store in an airtight container at room temperature for 3 days.

Chocolate-Covered Coconut Macaroons

Ingredients :

- 3 large egg whites
- ¼ teaspoon cream of tartar
- ⅛ teaspoon salt
- ¼ teaspoon pure almond extract
- ½ cup granulated sugar
- ⅔ cup gluten-free all-purpose flour with xanthan gum
- 4 cups sweetened shredded coconut
- 1½ cups gluten-free and dairy-free chocolate chips
- 2 teaspoons coconut oil melted

Directions :

1. Preheat oven to 350°F degrees and line two baking sheets with parchment paper.

2. In a large bowl, use a mixer to beat egg whites, cream of tartar, and salt until foamy. Add almond extract. Add sugar 1 tablespoon at a time and continue to beat. Add flour 1 tablespoon at a time and continue to beat until stiff. Stir in shredded coconut.

3. Scoop out dough using a 1½-tablespoons cookie scoop and place on prepared baking sheets.

4. Bake for 18–20 minutes until the cookie edges start to turn golden brown. Remove from the oven and allow cookies to cool completely before dipping them in chocolate.

5. In a microwave-safe dish, melt chocolate chips for 1–2 minutes, then stir and continue microwaving 30 seconds at a time until chips melt and are smooth. Once chocolate chips are fully melted, add coconut oil and stir. Dip the top of each cookie into the melted chocolate. Allow chocolate to cool for 1–2 minutes before serving cookies. Store in an airtight container at room temperature for up to 3 days.

Easy Gluten-Free Chocolate Cake with Chocolate Buttercream Frosting

Ingredients :

CAKE
- 1 cup unsweetened almond milk
- 1 tablespoon white vinegar
- 2 cups gluten-free all-purpose flour with xanthan gum
- 1 teaspoon salt
- 1 teaspoon baking soda
- ½ teaspoon gluten-free baking powder
- ½ teaspoon ground cinnamon
- ½ cup plus 1 tablespoon dairy-free buttery spread, softened

- 2 cups granulated sugar
- 2 large eggs
- 1 teaspoon pure vanilla extract
- ¾ cup cocoa powder
- ¾ cup boiling water

CHOCOLATE BUTTERCREAM FROSTING
- 1 cup dairy-free buttery spread
- 2 teaspoons pure vanilla extract
- ¼ teaspoon pure almond extract
- 1 cup cocoa powder
- ⅛ teaspoon salt
- 4 cups confectioners' sugar
- 3 tablespoons unsweetened almond milk

Directions :

1. Preheat oven to 350°F degrees. Cut parchment paper for the bottom of two 8" cake pans and spray with gluten-free nonstick cooking spray.
2. In a small bowl, combine milk and vinegar and allow to sit for 5 minutes to make buttermilk.
3. In a medium bowl, stir together flour, salt, baking soda, baking powder, and cinnamon.
4. In a large bowl, beat buttery spread and sugar together on medium speed until smooth.
5. Add eggs and vanilla extract to the buttery spread mixture and mix until fully combined.
6. Add the flour mixture to the buttery spread mixture and mix until fully combined.
7. Add the milk mixture to the buttery spread mixture and mix until fully combined.
8. Add cocoa powder to batter and mix until fully combined.
9. Add boiling water to batter and mix until fully combined.
10. 10 Divide batter evenly between prepared cake pans.
11. Bake on the middle rack for 30–35 minutes or until a toothpick inserted in the center comes out clean and the side of cake is pulling away from the side of the pan.
12. 12 Cool cakes in the pans for about 10–15 minutes. Then use a knife to loosen cakes around the edges of the pans and invert cakes onto a cooling rack to completely cool before frosting.
13. 13 In a large bowl, beat buttery spread at medium speed until smooth. Add vanilla and almond extracts and mix until fully combined.
14. 14 Add the cocoa powder and salt and mix until fully combined.
15. 15 Add confectioners' sugar 1 cup at a time and mix until fully combined.
16. 16 Add milk and beat until smooth and spreadable. Spread frosting between layers of cake and cover

top and sides. Store leftovers in an airtight container for up to 3 days.

Chocolate Peanut Butter Brownies

Ingredients :
- ½ cup dairy-free buttery spread, melted
- 1 tablespoon pure vanilla extract
- ¾ cup granulated sugar
- ½ cup light brown sugar, packed
- 2 large eggs, room temperature
- ¾ cup gluten-free all-purpose flour with xanthan gum
- ½ cup cocoa powder
- ½ teaspoon baking soda
- ½ teaspoon salt
- ¼ cup gluten-free peanut butter

Directions :

1. Preheat oven to 350°F and line an 8" × 8" baking pan with parchment paper and coat the bottom and sides with gluten-free nonstick cooking spray or buttery spread.

2. In a large bowl, add buttery spread, vanilla extract, granulated sugar, and brown sugar and mix until fully combined.

3. Add in eggs one at a time and mix until fully combined.

4. In a medium bowl, stir together flour, cocoa powder, baking soda, and salt.

5. Slowly add the flour mixture to the buttery spread mixture and mix until fully combined and smooth.

6. Pour the brownie batter into prepared baking pan. Drop 6 tablespoons of peanut butter on top of brownie batter in two rows of three. Take a knife and drag it through peanut butter and brownie batter to make a swirl pattern.

7. Bake for 30–35 minutes or until a toothpick inserted in the center comes out just barely clean and the sides of brownies start to pull away from the pan. Let brownies cool completely, about 30 minutes, in the pan before slicing. Store in an airtight at room temperature container for up to 3 days.

Frosted Coconut Cake

Ingredients :

CAKE
- ⅔ cup dairy-free buttery spread
- 1⅔ cups granulated sugar
- 1 teaspoon pure almond extract

- 2¼ cups gluten-free all-purpose flour with xanthan gum
- 3½ teaspoons gluten-free baking powder
- ½ teaspoon salt
- 1½ cups unsweetened coconut milk beverage (carton)
- 2 cups sweetened shredded coconut
- 5 large egg whites

FROSTING
- 1 cup dairy-free buttery spread, softened
- 1½ teaspoons pure vanilla extract
- ¼ teaspoon pure almond extract
- 4 cups confectioners' sugar
- 1 cup sweetened shredded coconut

Directions :

1. Preheat oven to 350°F. Cut parchment paper for the bottom of two 8" cake pans and spray with gluten-free nonstick cooking spray.
2. In a large bowl, beat together buttery spread and sugar on medium speed until smooth. Add almond extract and mix to combine. Add flour, baking powder, and salt and mix until fully combined. Add the coconut milk and shredded coconut and mix until fully combined.
3. Beat in egg whites and mix on high for 2 minutes.
4. Divide batter evenly between prepared cake pans.
5. Bake on the middle rack for 23–28 minutes or until a toothpick inserted in the center comes out clean and the sides of the cake are pulling away from the sides of the pan.
6. In a large bowl, beat buttery spread at medium speed until smooth. Add vanilla and almond extracts. Mix until fully combined.
7. Add confectioners' sugar 1 cup at a time to the buttery spread mixture and mix until fully combined.
8. Add coconut and mix until fully combined.
9. Cool cakes in the pans for about 10–15 minutes. Then use a knife to loosen cakes around the edges of the pans and invert cakes onto a cooling rack to completely cool before frosting. Spread frosting between layers of cake and cover top and sides. Store in an airtight container for up to 3 days.

Cinnamon Roll Cookies

Ingredients :

COOKIES
- ½ cup dairy-free buttery spread
- ½ cup light brown sugar, packed

- ¼ cup sugar
- 2 large eggs
- 2 teaspoons pure vanilla extract
- 2½ cups plus 1 tablespoon gluten-free all-purpose flour with xanthan gum, divided
- 1 teaspoon gluten-free baking powder
- ½ teaspoon baking soda
- ¼ teaspoon salt

FILLING

- ¼ cup light brown sugar, packed
- 1 tablespoon ground cinnamon

GLAZE

- ¼ cup light brown sugar, packed
- 3 tablespoons dairy-free buttery spread, melted
- 1 cup confectioners' sugar
- 1 tablespoon unsweetened almond milk

Directions :

1. In a large bowl, beat together buttery spread, brown sugar, and granulated sugar at medium speed until smooth.

2. Add eggs and vanilla extract and mix until fully combined. In a medium bowl, stir together 2½ cups flour, baking powder, baking soda, and salt. Pour the flour mixture into the buttery spread mixture and mix until fully combined.

3. Sprinkle remaining 1 tablespoon flour on a piece on parchment paper. Remove cookie dough from the bowl and shape it into a ball.

4. Form dough round about 7" in diameter and 1" thick.

5. Mix brown sugar and cinnamon together in a small bowl. Pour the mixture over cookie dough and pat down lightly.

6. Roll dough into a log shape. Wrap log in parchment paper, place on a baking sheet, and refrigerate for 1 hour.

7. Preheat oven to 375°F and line two baking sheets with parchment paper.

8. Using a knife or a pastry scraper, cut dough into ½" slices. Carefully put cookie slices on prepared baking sheets about 2" apart. Bake cookies for 10–12 minutes until golden around the edges.

9. In a small bowl, stir together brown sugar and buttery spread. Add confectioners' sugar and stir until it starts to thicken. Add milk to thin out glaze. Drizzle glaze all over the cookies, just like a cinnamon roll. Allow cookies to cool for 2–3 minutes before moving to cooling rack.

Apple Pie Blondies

Ingredients :

FILLING
- 1 tablespoon dairy-free buttery spread
- 2 cups peeled and diced Red Delicious apples
- 2 tablespoons light brown sugar, packed
- 1 teaspoon ground cinnamon
- 1 teaspoon pure vanilla extract

BLONDIE
- ½ cup dairy-free buttery spread, softened
- ¾ cup light brown sugar, packed
- 2 large eggs
- 1 tablespoon pure vanilla extract
- 1½ cups gluten-free all-purpose flour with xanthan gum
- 1 teaspoon gluten-free baking powder
- 1 teaspoon ground cinnamon
- ⅛ teaspoon ground nutmeg
- ½ teaspoon salt

GLAZE
- 1 cup confectioners' sugar
- 3 tablespoons pure maple syrup
- 1 teaspoon pure vanilla extract

Directions :

1. Preheat oven to 350°F and line an 8" × 8" baking pan with parchment paper and coat with gluten-free nonstick cooking spray.

2. In a small saucepan, add buttery spread, apples, brown sugar, cinnamon, and vanilla extract. Cook over medium heat for 1–2 minutes until buttery spread is melted. Stir diced apples to fully coat. Allow the mixture to come to a slight boil. Cook for 2–3 minutes until apples are soft and remove from the heat.

3. In a large bowl, beat buttery spread and brown sugar together on medium speed until smooth. Add eggs and vanilla extract and mix until fully combined.

4. Add flour, baking powder, cinnamon, nutmeg, and salt and mix until ingredients are fully combined. The blondie batter will be sticky.

5. Pour batter into prepared pan. Pour apple filling on top of blondie batter and spread to cover evenly.

6. Bake for 35–45 minutes until golden brown. The sides on the blondies will start to pull away from the sides of the pan.

7. Allow blondies to cool for 1 hour before adding glaze.
8. In a small bowl, stir together the glaze ingredients until smooth. Drizzle glaze on top of warm blondies.
9. Remove blondies from the pan by carefully lifting them up with the parchment paper. Refrigerate in an airtight container up to 3 days.

Peanut Butter Blossoms

Ingredients :

COOKIES
- ½ cup granulated sugar
- ½ cup light brown sugar, packed
- ½ cup dairy-free buttery spread
- ½ cup gluten-free peanut butter
- 1 large egg
- 1 teaspoon molasses
- 1¼ cups gluten-free all-purpose flour with xanthan gum
- ¾ teaspoon baking soda
- ½ teaspoon gluten-free baking powder
- ¼ cup granulated sugar for rolling

DAIRY-FREE CHOCOLATE PEANUT BUTTER FILLING
- ¾ cup gluten-free peanut butter
- 4 tablespoons cocoa powder
- 1 tablespoon pure vanilla extract
- ¾ cup confectioners' sugar
- 5 tablespoons unsweetened almond milk

Directions :

1. In a large bowl, beat together granulated sugar, brown sugar, buttery spread, and peanut butter at medium speed until fully combined and creamy. Mix in egg and molasses until combined.
2. In a medium bowl, stir together flour, baking soda, and baking powder.
3. Slowly pour the flour mixture into batter and mix until fully combined. The cookie dough will be like soft Play-Doh.
4. Cover cookie dough and refrigerate for 30 minutes.
5. Preheat oven to 375°F and line two baking sheets with parchment paper. Add ¼ cup granulated sugar to a small bowl. Scoop tablespoonfuls of dough and roll into balls with your hands. Roll balls in granulated sugar and place onto prepared baking sheets.

6. Bake for 10–12 minutes or until light brown on the edges.

7. As soon as you bring cookies out of the oven, use the back of a rounded teaspoon to make an indent in the center of the cookie. Allow cookies to cool for 2–3 minutes before moving to a cooling rack. Cool completely before adding filling.

8. In a large bowl, mix together the peanut butter, cocoa powder, and vanilla extract until fully combined. Add confectioners' sugar and mix until combined. Add milk and mix until smooth. Either pipe or spoon filling into the centers of cookies. Store in an airtight container at room temperature for up to 3 days.

Printed in Great Britain
by Amazon